MIDLIFE AT ST. MARGARET'S

Midlife at St. Margaret's

A Derivative Work of (Peri)Menopausal Brainfog

KATE BLANCHARD

Because Why Not

Contents

✳

— Dante Alighieri, 1472,
The Divine Comedy

— Judy Blume, 1970,
Are You There, God? It's Me, Margaret.

Chapter 1

Moving Day

We moved on the Tuesday before Labor Day, exactly one week after my husband of 22 years announced he was leaving.

With my almost-8th-grader at her bestie's for one last sleepover and my almost-senior sequestered in his room, I had spent Monday night alone on a deflating air mattress. I worked on my laptop till my eyes stopped functioning and then slept fitfully for a few hours. I awoke, flat on the floor, with the cat stomping back and forth between my bladder and my boobs.

"Ugh, Fiona." She purred loudly and leaned in close, rubbing her head on my face. I brushed cat hair out of my nose and sat up with a groan, body silently screaming. *I already hate this day.* Remembering that I needed to be strong for my traumatized kids, I switched my inner monologue to the only pep talk I could muster: *Just do the thing and it will soon be over.* Then I felt guilty for wishing away my "one wild and precious life," in disobedience of Mary Oliver and the Instagram algorithm.

We had already said goodbye to my parents. "Why are you doing this to your kids?" my mother had asked. She didn't ask out loud how I could do this to her and my dad, but I knew that question was lurking in the background.

"Can't you just ask your boss to take you back? Or why don't you talk to Mildred's son? He's a dean at Columbia now, maybe he knows of a job for you." At that moment she looked so old, wiping her nose with a worn-out tissue. I hugged her.

"Mom, for the millionth time, that's not how academia works. Once you quit, they don't take you back. I'm lucky to have a job at all in this market."

In truth I felt horrible about leaving them. But I had to earn a living, and very few employers were clamoring for middle-aged white ladies with PhDs in Italian Renaissance literature. My old institution had barely waited a day after my departure before announcing they were cutting Italian altogether. Don't let the *porta* hit you on the way out.

The morning was a blur of wrangling two angry teens, packing up the cat and the remnants of our stuff into the overstuffed minivan, and tearfully locking the door of the only home my kids had ever known. By the time I settled into the driver's seat I was sweating profusely. I stripped down to my tank top and unconsciously sniffed my un-shaved armpits.

"Ew, Mom!" Kelsey said, taking a brief break from crying to disapprove.

We set out through the winding roads of our old neigh-borhood and headed to the interstate, waving goodbye to our favorite places, and finally to New Jersey. This set Kelsey off into a new fit of crying. "What if I hate my new school? What if everyone hates me?"

I assured her, again, that she had always had lots of friends and would make new friends in no time. About my firstborn in the back seat I was less certain, but he tended to keep his existential crises to himself.

When we crossed into our new home state, Kelsey snapped a picture of the "Welcome to Pure Michigan" sign and posted it immediately to her feeds. She was now thirteen, finally old enough for Instagram and Snapchat, and we had given her a smartphone for her birthday (which I almost immediately regretted, even though most of her friends had gotten them long before). We obeyed Siri for another couple of hours till we finally saw the exit for St. Jutta, which led us to a country road. On my first visit I had pronounced the name as if it were German, "YOU-ta," but I soon learned the locals called it "St. Judah."

"Who even is St. Jutta?" Kelsey shouted from beneath her headphones. I happened to know the answer because I had Googled it.

"St. Judith of Thuringia, patron saint of Prussia."

"Russia?"

"No, Prussia."

"Like the King of Prussia mall?"

"Um, yeah." St. Jutta was a hermit. I kind of envied her.

"Huh," she said. We passed a defunct oil refinery. "Where's the town?"

"It's just up ahead," I replied cheerfully. *Please be just up ahead*. I really had to pee. Again.

Soon enough, a brown sign said "College of St. Margaret, 2" with an arrow pointing past a patch of trees that provided a screen for yet another wide open field. Eliot, having made barely a peep for nine hours, began singing the dueling banjos from *Deliverance*.

I shared their misgivings. I, too, worried about everyone at my new school hating me. In addition, I worried—as I passed a homemade Trump billboard, not too long after the giant anti-abortion billboard and the barn with the Confederate battle flag painted on it—about raising my kids in what felt like a foreign country. A little roadside stand with a sign that said "Fresh Tomatos" and "CORN" made me feel a bit better with its farm kitschiness, spelling be damned.

We passed some warehouses, a cannabis dispensary (I made a mental note just in case), and a municipal building before coming to our first traffic light. A brick sign on one corner said, "Welcome to St. Jutta, a Great Place to Call Home." Also at the intersection were a gas station, a dollar store, and a storefront church that was also gun and pawn shop. On the next block a marquis announced an upcoming "St. Jutta's Got Talent" show.

Focus on the positive, Jen.

"Isn't it cute? It's just like something out of a movie."

"Yeah, if you like living in the Upside Down," Eliot said.

A couple of blocks later we left the main road and turned down a bumpy street made of bricks. I did some Kegels. "Guys, could you get Fiona back in her crate? We're almost there. For real this time."

We pulled into the driveway at 305 West Chapel Street, a brown bungalow with a big porch and an overgrown lawn. It was almost nine but still surprisingly light out, and the evening felt gloriously cool. The leaves high up in the trees were kind of whispering to each other, and I heard a lone cicada who had apparently missed his moment. *Dude, same.* Inside I made a beeline for the powder room, trying not to focus too hard on the stained chartreuse carpet, faded wallpaper, or musty old-person smell.

I could hear the kids stomping up the stairs to find their bedrooms. None of us had actually seen the house before, except in pictures. Moose, my soon-to-be-ex-husband, had come out alone in July and bought it, promising me it "had great bones." That was before the unthinkable happened. I was now in sole charge of home logistics for the first time in two decades and I didn't like it one bit. But since it couldn't be helped, I would put on my proverbial big-girl pants and be grateful they weren't yet Depends.

I awoke that night in a sweat, as usual, around 3:00 a.m. After wiping myself down with a cold washcloth, I crept into my kids' rooms to check on them, like when they were babies. Kelsey always abandoned herself to sleep, arms and legs extended, blankets in a tangle. Eliot slept like a corpse, on his back in a long, straight line, faintly snoring. Some-day he would probably snore like a chainsaw, like Moose did till he got a CPAP machine. After that, he insisted I get one too. *His and hers*, I used to joke. *So sexy*. I had resisted throwing my expensive machine in the dumpster before we left New Jersey, but I had no intention of using it while sleeping alone.

Chapter 2

How I Got Dumped

I suppose you need to know what happened with Moose and me. It's a tired cliché and utterly humiliating.

Moose—Matthew Joseph Miglione, Jr.—and I were one of those rare couples who were both born and raised in New Jersey, by parents who were also born and raised in New Jersey. I am from a moneyed suburb close to New York, he from a working-class neighborhood near Trenton. My family—the Smiths—are about as WASPy as it gets, but as a kid I always wanted to be Italian because the cool kids around me had the best last names—Colello, Bianculli, LaRusso, Marchesi. (I would have settled for Ferguson, Sullivan, O'Brien, or Murphy.)

Basically, Moose and I had bonded over Italy. We met in grad school. That is, *I* was in grad school, studying the Italian Renaissance at Princeton. He was a Princeton math alum working in the university's IT department. He was a Mac, I was a PC. I wrote most of my dissertation in my favorite local coffee shop, and once when it was really crowded, he asked if he could share my table. He was cute and nerdy and kinetic and funny and had a real job—a welcome relief from all my time spent among depressed (and broke) grad students.

I suppose he enjoyed the experience of sweeping someone serious off her feet. He took to greeting me with "*Buonjourno, principessa!*" after we saw *Life Is Beautiful*. We were both ambitious, but in ways that didn't compete with each other. We liked to take long drives—to Manhattan, Trenton, Philadelphia—to find the best Italian food, while dreaming out loud about our future. It was a bonus that I could actually talk to his grandma, who had come to the US as a young woman. We married late in 1999 and partied like...well, you know.

In 2001 I graduated with my PhD and we moved up to my alma mater, Madison College, where I got one of the country's last tenure-track jobs in Italian Language and Literature when my former professor retired. The 9/11 attacks happened in my first month as an assistant professor, so I can pretty much say teaching never got harder than that, at least until March 2020. We had Eliot before I got tenure and Kelsey after, with a couple of miscarriages in between. Moose wanted a third child but by then our lives were so busy, and I was so maxed out, that I didn't have it in me to keep trying. We had a boy, a girl, a house, two cars, two jobs, two sets of nearby in-laws—what more did we need?

After two decades we were well past our honeymoon, as boring as any happily married couple. Date nights were rare, sex even rarer. But we were still good friends, kind of like siblings. We fought sometimes—I got annoyed that he always seemed to have plenty of time for cycling or trivia nights with friends but not for dishes or home maintenance; he got annoyed that I worked all the time and was a nag. But mostly we got along and could count on each other to have our backs.

Or so I thought. I had certainly noticed some distance between us, and I fully expected our marriage to need some repair and renovation eventually, like a house with great bones that just needs a little TLC. But we had so much else going on that I figured it just wasn't time to focus on that yet. It seemed like a project for after the kids were out of the house. I guess I overestimated Moose's ability or willingness to wait that long.

When the pandemic started, his job went fully remote for several months, which he loved because it left him more time for cycling. In the fall of 2020, I was trying to teach Italian in half-empty college classrooms while wearing a mask, while simultaneously producing online lectures that could be streamed later by the rest of my sleepy or sick students. By then I was a full professor, as well as the half-time Dean of Arts and Humanities, which meant I was also trying to help manage the anxieties of my colleagues and keep the Vice President of Academic Affairs off their backs. It must be said that I failed spectacularly despite my best efforts: not only was my own major cut, but so were dance, religious studies, and every modern language except Spanish.

Anyway, though our marriage had slumped and sagged its way into a fixer-upper, Moose had always been a loving and involved dad. One of his favorite things was taking the kids somewhere fun on spring break, just the three of them, since the college never had the same break as the public schools. I always felt a little left out, but it made me happy to see my kids enjoy time with their father. In 2021 he splurged and took them to Costa Rica, which was all the rage with his coworkers. They did some sightseeing, snorkeling, and a whole lot of "laying out" (as Kelsey would say) on the beach or by the hotel pool.

The kids had fun, but apparently not as much fun as Moose.

Months later, after I had accepted a new job ("Come on," he said, "it'll be exciting! You need to move on from Madison University!") and he had bought us a new house, he decided to tell me about it.

"Jen, we need to talk." I was in our bathroom throwing miscellaneous toiletries into a box.

"Ok," I said, still packing.

"No, really, I need you to come in here and sit down."

My stomach lurched. "Who's dead?" I sat on the bed.

"No one's dead." That came as some relief, but my heart kept thumping as he sat down next to me. I tried to read the strange look on his face. He took a deep breath.

"I've met someone and I'm leaving."

I stared, not computing.

"Jen? Did you hear what I said?"

"You've met someone," I said robotically. "You're leaving." Over his shoulder, I could see Eliot's old crayon marks on the wall. *I should clean those off before we move.*

He took a breath and tried again. "I've fallen in love with another woman and I'm leaving you and moving in with her." I stared down at my hands. A France-shaped age spot had taken up residence above my left thumb.

"Jen? Aren't you going to say anything?"

When I didn't, he stood up and started pacing. "See this is why I'm leaving. You have no emotions. You never react to anything like a normal person!"

That snapped me out of it. "I'm processing," I said, looking him in the eyes. "Are you seriously yelling at me right now for processing?"

"You aren't even reacting! I've just told you I'm divorcing you, and you're not doing anything! You're not yelling, you're not crying, nothing!" His arms waved in exasperation. My perceived lack of feelings had been a sore point between us almost since the beginning. Opposites attract, but they also drive each other crazy.

My chest and neck felt hot. "I honestly don't know how to react, Moose. I'm still trying to figure out if this is real."

"It's real. I'm leaving you. Tomorrow. Forever. For real."

The words hung in the air.

"Who is she?" I finally had the wherewithal to ask.

"Amber."

"Amber?" I repeated. "From work?" He nodded. "I thought she moved to Costa Rica because of Covid..." A lightbulb went on and something slowly formed itself in my brain. "Did it start over spring break?"

He winced. "No. It started a couple of years ago, and then it stopped when she moved to Costa Rica. But we... kept in touch."

The inside of my head buzzed like a swarm of bees. My ears were ringing. The room seemed to expand and contract in slow motion.

"So," I said slowly, by the force of sheer will, "you're leaving me...and our children...and moving to another country...to be with someone you've been having an affair with for a couple of years."

He sighed and his arms dropped to his sides. "Yes."

"And you waited to tell me this until after I quit my job, and just a few days before we uprooted our children from everything and everyone they know." I looked at my puffy finger outgrowing its wedding band.

"I know," he started pacing again, "but they'll be fine. Eliot's almost out of the house anyway, and Kelsey still has you."

"What the hell is that supposed to mean, *she still has me?*"

"I mean, she's a girl and she mostly needs her mother."

I stood up. "Are you out of your mind?"

"What?" he asked, indignant. "It'll be great. They loved Costa Rica and they can visit me on breaks. It will expand their world. They can learn Spanish. You always complain that American kids don't learn foreign languages!"

I began to shake and realized I needed a toilet immediately. I headed for the bathroom.

"That's right," he shouted, "walk away like you always do."

I whipped around to face him. "I HAVE TO GO TO THE TOILET AND YOU'RE THE ONE LEAVING WITHOUT SO MUCH AS A WARNING! JESUS CHRIST, MOOSE!"

"What's going on?" Kelsey stood in the doorway.

"Ask your father," I said petulantly. I didn't want to leave but I was literally about to lose my shit. I hurried into the bathroom, managed to close the door without slamming it, and sat down. "I'll be right there, Kels," I shouted. Muffled through the door I could hear them having almost the same exchange he and I had just had. *When did my life become a bad sitcom?*

"I hate you!" She finally screamed. I heard our bedroom door slam, and then a few seconds later her bedroom door.

"Aw honey, don't cry," I heard Moose say, moving out into the hallway. I heard a faint knocking on her door, Moose pleading with Kelsey to open it. I cleaned myself up, washed my hands, and followed them. Moose stood forlorn at his daughter's locked door, looking at me with pleading eyes. By now Eliot was also standing silently in his doorway, somewhere between alarmed and annoyed.

"Let me," I said quietly. "Go talk to your son."

Moose obeyed, and I called to Kelsey through the door. Eventually she opened it, red eyed and confused and so damn vulnerable.

"Mom?" she said, starting to sob again. I took her into my arms.

"I know, hon," I said, "it's gonna be ok."

Is it going to be ok? I asked myself. *Yes, it has to be.*

Chapter 3

First Day of School

So here I was in Michigan without a husband.

On Wednesday morning, after another stupid night on the air mattress, I made a quick trip to the grocery store before the movers arrived. The town of St. Jutta was small and the roads almost empty. The nearest grocery was a big box store called Meijer, apparently Michigan's version of Target or Walmart. The right half was groceries, and the left half was everything else. I hadn't planned any meals so I picked up some essentials—coffee, eggs, bread, milk, bananas, chicken breasts, veggie burgers, pasta, cat food, and cat litter—just until I could get my act together. Keeping us alive was my new bar for success.

When I got home Kelsey was sitting on the porch swing eating a doughnut and looking at her phone.

"Hey, where'd you get that?" I asked, leaning over to kiss the top of her head, resenting the way my jeans cut into my midriff.

"Some lady brought them over," she answered with a mouthful.

"Some lady?"

"Mmm hmm."

"Who?"

"I dunno, Eliot talked to her," she shrugged toward the house. "She has a pool!"

I carried the bags into the kitchen, where Eliot was leaning with his back against the counter, also eating a doughnut and looking at his phone. I greeted him as I put the bags on the counter next to him. I got no reaction so I greeted him again more loudly.

"What?" he frowned.

"Who brought the doughnuts?" I asked as pleasantly as I could. He was no longer a morning person. Even late morning. Or, you know, any time of day when his mother could be seen or heard.

"I dunno, some lady from across the street. There's a note." He tipped his chin toward a white bakery box on the counter.

"Huh. Well that was nice of her. How are you doing this morning?"

"Fine."

I stared at him a moment too long, knowing he must still be in pain about his dad. I wanted more than anything to hug him, and he must have sensed this because he fled the kitchen just as Fiona came to investigate.

I scratched the cat's backside and grabbed a doughnut from the box. It felt cakey and firm, more Dunkin' than Krispy Kreme, but less mass-produced. I bit into it and a sprinkling of crunchy cinnamon sugar fell onto my chest.

"Oh my god, that's good," I said out loud, gobbling it down.

The envelope next to it read "New Neighbors" in elegant cursive. Inside was a notecard with a T-Rex wearing sunglasses, shooting a rainbow out of its mouth. Inside it read, "Welcome to the neighborhood! Please reach out if you need anything. Enjoy the best doughnuts in Michigan! —Jamie Schroeder at #308." Her phone number and email address were also there.

As I reached for a second doughnut (*Savor it this time, Jen*), I made a mental note to go thank her after the movers had come and gone this afternoon. I wandered back into the living room, where through the front window I could see my kids sitting together in companionable silence on the porch swing. We didn't have any other chairs yet, so I just sat in the middle of the living room floor. After I finished eating I lay down and stared at the ceiling, trying not to freak out about everything I had to do.

That night, after somehow surviving the controlled chaos of the movers, we all went to bed in real beds, surrounded by boxes. The next morning was a big day—my first day at the office and my first meeting with the president's cabinet —so I hoped to get a good night's sleep. Instead, I tossed and turned in my half empty queen, unable to shut my brain up or my internal heater off. I turned on my favorite linguistics podcast and kind of faded in and out. At some point, I snored myself awake and realized one episode had ended and another one had started. I turned it off and finally slept for a few hours.

My mom called the next morning as I was searching through boxes for the coffee maker, cursing last night's Jen for not having done it before she went to bed. Normally I would have thought of this but I wasn't quite myself.

"Hi, hon," she said.

"Hi, Ma," I said distractedly, "how's it going?" I put her on speaker so I could open another box.

"Well, Dad's in the hospital," she said.

"What?" I stopped still.

"He has a kidney infection from a UTI."

"Oh my God, Mom." I took the box off a chair and sat down. I heard her sigh. "What does that mean? Is he ok?"

"He's doing better this morning. He was in pretty bad shape yesterday." She sounded tired. "He's getting IV antibiotics." She greeted someone in the background.

"Why didn't you call me yesterday?" I was filled with shame for not checking in on them last night.

"Oh, I didn't want to bother you when you were dealing with the movers and everything."

"Mom! You should always call me about things like this!"

"Hon, can I call you back in a minute? I need to order Dad's lunch now." I rolled my eyes—this was often how phone calls with my mother went—but let her go with a sigh.

After I hung up a wave of guilt washed over me for abandoning them in their twilight years. *That's not helpful, Jen. Even you can't fix a UTI.* I shook it off and tried to remember what I had been doing. The automatic coffeemaker still eluded me but I found the French press and a soup pan so I boiled some water and made a pot. The water coming out of the tap smelled strongly of chlorine, but I didn't have time to worry about the cancer-causing oxidants I was putting in my body, or the fact that I now lived in the same state as Flint.

Back in my room, I took off my sweaty bedclothes and hung them on a curtain rod to dry (after making sure my window faced the back yard rather than the street or a neighbor's window). I tried out my new shower before remembering I didn't yet know where my towels were, so I dried off with a sheet.

Still damp, I cursed while struggling into my bra and the torture device designed to hold in my expanding lower body, euphemistically known as "shapewear." I hadn't worn anything but tank tops and leggings or lounge pants for the past two months (ok fine, two years) so this felt even more insulting than usual, but it couldn't be helped. I made a mental note to order some bigger clothes—again—as soon as possible.

Once upon a time, I liked getting dressed up for work. While in Italy, I had acquired an appreciation for fashion and high-quality clothing. Maybe it was a cliché, but wearing nice things made me feel more powerful, especially as a young professor. But as my body had grown wider in the last few years, dressing up had gotten less and less fun. Clothes had begun stretching in multiple places, instead of falling comfortably like they used to. I now got dressed out of a sense of duty, more like a uniform than armor. I never felt beautiful, but I could at least relax a little bit if I knew I was dressed appropriately.

I put on some makeup and sighed at my drooping neck, which had absorbed my chin seemingly overnight in my late 40s. *They hired you for your brains, not your looks*, I told myself. *Anyway, it all makes you look less intimidating.*

It was just before 8:00 a.m. when I left. The kids were still sleeping, so I sent them a text reminding them of my whereabouts and that there was food in the fridge. The day would grow hot but wasn't yet, and I enjoyed my walk to campus, most of which was in the shade of big old trees. In a yard with a Trump 2020 sign (the second zero had been crossed out and replaced it with a four), there was also one that said, "My Governor Is An Idiot." *I guess it's kinder than a similar slogan in New Jersey would be.*

All in all, my new commute felt like a gift compared to the competitive driving event that was my old commute, where I had to channel my inner Imperator Furiosa. It took all of about four minutes to get from my front door to the dragon-bedecked entry gate that welcomed me to the central quad of the College of St. Margaret.

The school was named for Margaret of Antioch, sometimes called Margaret the Virgin, who stood in stone form just beyond the main gate, a book in one hand and a weapon in the other that was somewhere between a sword and a cross. She was also known as St. Marina, the Great Martyr and Vanquisher of Demons, tortured and murdered back in the day for refusing to get married and make babies like a good Roman girl. Before being relieved of her head, she was swallowed and fought her way out of the belly of Satan in the form of a dragon. About a thousand years later she hung out in spirit with another famous virgin, Joan of Arc.

Despite her own virginity, Margaret ended up becoming a patron saint of all things birth related—expectant mothers, nursing mothers, and those in labor—perhaps because her own mother died in childbirth. *What can you do for single mothers of teenagers?* In any case, a dragon-vanquishing virgin struck me as a pretty cool mascot for a Catholic women's college. It wasn't all women anymore—it had gone coed in the seventies in its attempt to stay afloat, and the football team alone now accounted for about a tenth of the student body. If not for Division III sports, small private colleges would almost certainly have gone extinct by now.

I hadn't actually been back to St. Margaret's or St. Jutta since February of 2020, when I flew out to interview for the provost job. At the time the whole place looked gray. There had been patches of dirty, crusty snow on the ground, the trees had been bare, and the sun never seemed to rise fully. So the sunny green lushness of late summer came as a welcome surprise. In normal times I, as an incoming provost, would have gotten the job months ago, and would have already been making regular visits to the college through the spring and summer to start planning with the president and his cabinet. But I had not gotten the job under normal circumstances.

In fact, I didn't even get the job to begin with, despite making it to the short list. In 2020, it had instead gone to a hotshot younger guy (by which I mean early forties). But, somehow, even in the midst of social distancing and online meetings, he had managed to harass no fewer than three junior faculty women in less than a year. One of them told her department chair, a second-wave feminist, who started asking around till she found two more of his victims and then made a formal complaint to the president. The president promised to give the provost a firm talking-to, but begged the professor not to rock the boat because he was still brand new and the board really liked him.

Having none of it, the department chair went to the Title IX coordinator, and then to the director of HR, who eventually forced the president's hand—sort of. The provost was allowed to resign and leave quietly after his commencement duties. Before leaving, he had already secured a sweet new gig in fundraising at the national headquarters of his fraternity.

Anyway, given the extraordinary circumstances—the last guy's very short time on the job, the desperate need for someone (preferably a woman) to manage the faculty, and everyone's pandemic exhaustion—the board and president of St. Margaret's had decided not to start a new search from scratch, but instead go back into the short list of 2020, on which I was their second choice.

I got the call from President Norman Festerling in June of 2021, and he wanted an answer right away. When I had originally applied for the job, way back in the fall of 2019 (because academia moves about as quickly as molasses), Moose and I had both been more enthusiastic about moving. I was bored at work and couldn't fathom another 20 years of teaching, so shifting toward administration seemed the next natural step. Moose had never lived anywhere but New Jersey and said he wanted an adventure. He had also become grumpy about his job of late, although he could never quite express why. Looking back, I guess it's possible he felt guilty and thought getting away from Amber would save our marriage.

When the offer came out of the blue only about eight weeks ago, conditions at home had changed significantly. I was still bored and even more desperate to leave teaching after three semesters of Zoom, watching more and more students drop out or fail classes due to anxiety, depression, or general ennui. But Moose, who had encouraged me for years to move on from Madison, suddenly had no enthusiasm for moving. He pulled out every objection he could think of, starting with the kids. They were a year older, and moving them now would be cruel. I countered that Kelsey was an extrovert and still in middle school, so she had plenty of time to bounce back.

Eliot was...another story. If Kelsey was our dandelion child, he was our orchid, definitely not blooming where he was planted. Starting a new high school as a senior would certainly be difficult, but he was doing poorly in school anyway, and basically had no in-real-life friends or social life other than cross country. He could play his video games anywhere. Plus, I said, this job was an investment in their future; it almost doubled my salary, and the cost of living was much less than New Jersey, so we could finally get a bigger house and still have money to save.

Then, last but not least, Moose reminded me—as if I could forget—that I was an only child and my parents needed me. But they were both doing pretty well in their late 70s, still playing golf and taking their nightly "post-prandial" walks. I figured I would spend about five years in Michigan, just to get my feet wet as an administrator and get Kelsey through high school, and then I could get a better job back east and be there in time for their dotage.

After two sleepless nights, talks with my parents and boss, and an extended cold shoulder from Moose, I was planning to turn down the job. But he unexpectedly came home from work with renewed energy, urging me to take the job, determined to help the move go smoothly. I guess I should have been suspicious when his mood changed so quickly, but I had so many things to wrap up at my old job, plus getting our house cleaned up and on the market, that I just felt grateful.

Most unusually, because he wasn't typically proactive when it came to our domestic arrangements, he offered to take on the house-hunting by himself. I briefly hesitated—we had always made big decisions like that together—but since I was pushing him to move against his will, I thought letting him choose the house for us would help him feel better about things. So less than a month before, Moose had picked out the house we now lived in without him.

In hindsight, I was tortured by what ifs. *What if I had not taken the job? What if I had paid more attention to how weird he was being? What if I had put my kids and parents before my professional aspirations?* But that was pointless now.

So here I was, entering Bloom Hall, a building I had visited only once, a year and a half ago. Like most of the buildings on campus, it was more or less a big box made of red brick, built in the 1960s. The only exceptions I had noticed were the new athletics building (thanks to generous male alumni) and the one old stone building that had survived all the fires and improvements over the years, which held the offices of the president, CFO, COO, and VP for advancement.

I put on my mask as I approached the building. I was already sweating from my walk, and as I opened the door my heart started racing from the adrenaline of this new beginning. The air conditioning inside offered some relief and I paused for a moment to collect myself. The provost's office was on the ground floor, amid lecture halls and a computer lab. To get to my office, I had to pass through a little bay where the secretary's—or rather "office associate's"—desk was. There was also a small conference room off to one side. A plump white woman with fluffy salt-and-pepper hair, who looked a few years older than I, sat facing the door behind a large monitor on an L-shaped desk.

"Good morning, Fran!" I said a bit too loudly, trying to sound non-threatening.

Fran wasn't wearing a mask so I pulled mine off, afraid of seeming unfriendly or judgmental. She gave me a lukewarm "Hi" and then stared at me. I realized I hadn't plucked my newly-aggressive mustache hairs in a while and hoped that wasn't what she was looking at.

"It's good to see you in person again," I blustered. "Thanks so much for all your help the past few weeks." I had been emailing her furiously for all kinds of information and she had responded consistently, if without flourish. I suspected she was the real power broker around here and I wanted her to like me.

"Well, it's my job," she said. Her hand had never left her mouse. I waited to see if she would say anything else, so she finally asked, "How was your move?"

"Thanks, it was fine! It only took about eleven hours and my teenagers barely spoke the whole way so I got to listen to a bunch of good podcasts, in between my cat's yowls!" I made a little nervous laugh but she did not. *Too much information, Jen, take a breath. And stop yelling.*

"These are for you from President Festerling," said Fran flatly, finally letting go of her mouse to hand me a vase of flowers from her desk. They were mostly the nondescript purple filler kind, with a few white roses and daisies in the mix. A big blue and red ribbon was tied around the neck of the vase. For a second I thought it was being patriotic, before I remembered images of Margaret the Virgin dressed in her blue gown and red robe.

"How nice, thank you so much!" I was shouting again. *Take a damn breath.* "I'll put them on my desk." I looked toward the door to my office. It was closed and I didn't have a key so I stood there dumbly, my briefcase in one hand, flowers in the other.

"Oh, here," Fran said, standing up. "It's been cleaned." She opened the office door, which wasn't locked, and turned on the overhead lights, which made me wince. I put down my things on the large wooden desk against the wall and turned on a small desk lamp for some relief. There were bookshelves on two of the other walls, a wobbly desk chair on wheels, and one large leather chair in the corner.

"Your key's on the desk," she said. "Would you like some coffee?"

"I would LOVE some coffee!" *So much for gravitas.*

"It's in the lounge. I'll show you."

I followed her a short way down the main corridor, past an elevator to a mail room, behind which was the faculty lounge. It was a small, windowless room with a round table and a few chairs, a sink with three dirty mugs in it (a sign above it read, "PLEASE WASH YOUR OWN DISHES THERE IS NO MAID"), and a counter with a coffee maker, some clean mugs, and a stack of Styrofoam cups. *Who still uses Styrofoam?* I made a mental note to eliminate those as soon as possible.

"I just made it a few minutes ago." Fran gestured toward some (presumably) clean cups. "You can use one of these if you want." I picked a mug that said "Harvard" on it and then immediately wished I hadn't. What if this was a test, and I was giving off the impression of being elitist? I needed to distract her from my faux pas.

"So how long have you worked at St. Margaret's?"

"Thirty-two years," she said. "I started out working in the business office when my husband was a student and then just kept on working here." She paused so I could marvel inarticulately. "But I've only been in the provost's office for the last thirteen years." *Only?* I thought. *I hope I can last five.* As if reading my mind she said, "You're my fourth provost."

"Well I'm definitely going to rely on you for a lot of help while I'm getting up to speed." I was afraid that might have sounded threatening, so I added, with another laugh, "I mean I hardly know anything about this school *or* about being a provost!" I realized too late that did not sound reassuring.

She pursed her lips in disapproval before managing to bring her face back to its neutral position. Leading me back toward the office, she pointed out the closest bathroom, a unisex one-seater, as well as the bigger women's room down the hall that the students also used. I made mental notes of both in case of emergencies, and then decided to stop and use the one-seater preemptively. The last thing I needed was a leak on my first day at work that would follow me for the rest of my time here. Provost Pee Pee, I imagined as I sat. The Pissing Provost. *God, you're weird. And basic.*

The rest of the morning was a flurry of setting up my computer with IT, getting my picture taken for a new ID (*who is that fat old woman?*), meeting the librarians, and finally stopping by the president's office up on the third floor, to let him know I was ready for business. I greeted his executive assistant with as much professionalism as I could muster. She reminded me that he wasn't in that day; he was in Hilton Head on a fundraising mission. I had known this yesterday and completely forgotten, so it came as a great relief.

What I really wanted was to go home and take a nap, but there was still so much to do, so I headed back to my office. I told Fran I'd be working and closed my office door so I could put my head down on my desk for a few minutes.

Chapter 4

The Women's Caucus

I wouldn't have taken a lunch break at all, except I already had a scheduled meeting with the Faculty Women's Caucus—a meeting I'd forgotten about entirely until Fran knocked on my door.

"Your 11:45 is here," she said. I had no idea where I was or how long I'd been sleeping. I wiped the drool from the side of my mouth.

"My 11:45?"

"Joanne James? From sociology?"

It still didn't ring a bell but I nodded anyway. My neck was killing me. "OK thanks, I'll be right out."

When she left, closing the door behind her, I pulled up my calendar. Sure enough, the words "Faculty Women's Caucus?" were written there. *Shit.* I remembered someone—I thought her name was Vivian—had invited me a week or so ago, back when I still had a husband, to meet with them over lunch when I arrived. I had put it on my calendar and promptly forgotten all about it.

I got a mirror out of my bag and looked at my face to make sure all the crusties were gone. I ran my fingers through my hair, trying to cover up the big red mark on my forehead where I'd leaned on the desk, and hoped it was good enough.

When I walked out into the bay to greet Joanne I instinctually analyzed her appearance. This is something I always do and I *hate hate hate* it about myself, but I can't help it. Moose always called me out for it, and I knew it was wrong, but the beauty myth was stained into the fabric of my being before I was old enough to know it was happening. Try as I might, I couldn't seem to wash it out completely. I decided she was about my age and about my size, which put me at ease.

"Fran, I'll be back in an hour or so," I said.

"Uh-huh." Did I detect some irony in her tone, or was I just projecting?

Joanne offered to drive me in her giant SUV.

"I know it's a gas-guzzler," she said as we climbed in, "but we have three kids and two dogs and we just don't fit in anything smaller." Left-leaning academics are wont to both guilt and self-justification, even unprompted. The critics in our heads never shut up.

"I understand completely," I said. "I drive an old minivan, which isn't much better."

We chatted about our kids for all of ninety seconds before parking in front of a café called Grandma's that had a neon sign and other retro diner vibes. The writing on the door said "breakfast anytime we're open," and they were open daily from 7 a.m. to 2 p.m. (a mere shadow of the 24-hour Greek diners I was used to, but I guessed the customer base was a lot smaller here). There were also two other temporary signs, printed on office paper and taped to the door. One said masks were required for the unvaccinated, per current state guidelines. The other said the pandemic had made supply chains slow and politely asked customers not to be dicks about menu items that might not be available. I couldn't imagine how hard their last year and a half had been.

Inside, the air conditioning was on full blast and the retro vibes continued. There was an old soda-fountain-style bar to one side, with spinning vinyl stools, cracked from long use by the butts of St. Jutta. *No pie for you today, Madame Provost*, I said as I eyed a glass case with pies in it. I was surprised when Joanne led me to a booth near the back. I had assumed the Faculty Women's Caucus at a former women's college might be roughly half the faculty, so I expected a large crowd, but there turned out to be just three more white ladies sitting there, with a single chair pulled up at the end of the table.

Joanne sat down in the booth so I guessed the chair was for me. She introduced me to the others: Vivian, from the theater, art, and dance department (TAD); Barbara from the history, political science, philosophy, religion, and sociology department (HPPRS – they called it "hoppers"); and Elaine from the English and modern languages department (EML). All of them looked my age or older. Vivian was a ballet dancer, Elaine was a medieval historian, and Barbara specialized in 20th century Spanish literature. But since the school was so small, they, like pretty much all humanists, wore many hats and taught courses at best tangential to their specialties.

"It's so nice to meet you all," I said breathlessly, quickly adding "Again," in case we'd met before. I settled into my chair, scouting out the nearest rest room just in case. This was much more intimate than I had prepared myself for and I felt entirely frazzled and off balance. But since I was now the boss I thought it my job to put them at ease until they were ready to start in on their agenda. I hoped it was mostly informational rather than a request for money, because I hadn't had time to study the budgets yet.

"What can I get ya," said a tiny, gum-chewing woman of about 35 with a fluffy blondish ponytail, who bounced up next to me. My fellow diners seemed to be regulars because they all ordered without looking at their menus. Vivian and Joanne ordered house salads, Vivian with the raspberry vinaigrette and Joanne with Ranch. Elaine ordered a veggie burger with no bun and a side of cole slaw. And Barbara ordered a Reuben sandwich with fries and a milkshake. I was flustered so I ordered the house salad with vinaigrette (because all those beauty magazines I read in my teens said one should eat like the skinniest person at the table) and a diet coke.

I was sweating again. Or more accurately, still sweating. *Don't sniff your pits, Jen.*

"Thank you so much for joining us," said Vivian graciously. She was very wrinkled and very blonde, and even in the booth it was obvious she was tall. Despite a little hunch in her shoulders, she somehow still had posture that caused me to sit up straighter in my chair. "We are so glad to finally have a woman in the provost's office." The rest nodded in agreement.

I suddenly remembered Vivian from my campus interview two winters ago, because she had asked a question about "salary compression"—where older faculty end up being poorly compensated relative to their younger counterparts—after my presentation to the faculty. I had replied that of course there had to be pay equity among faculty members and was prepared to speak at some length about it, but I had cut my answer short when I noticed the president looking down uncomfortably.

That was only one of the several moments during that interview visit when I'd realized I said the wrong thing and thought, *There's no way you're getting this job.* It turned out I was right—but then none of us had counted on the other guy being a sexual predator. My being here was basically an overcorrection. In any case, the president was now stuck with an East Coast female provost who still thought like a professor. At least till I messed up and he could respectably send me on my way.

The four of them talked animatedly and nonstop for the next half-hour about all manner of women's issues on campus—bullying, unfair tenure denials, chair appointments, lack of childcare, inequitable service and advising loads—all things the president and the last two provosts apparently hadn't seen fit to address. But the biggest concern they had was salary inequity.

"We've talked to people privately, written memos to the provost and president, and debated it in committees," Barbara counted these items on her fingers and then threw up her hands and shrugged. "But most of the faculty are too scared to mobilize, and there's only so much a few of us can do if the administration isn't behind it."

"Totally," I said without thinking. As a faculty member I had banged my head against enough walls to know she was right. There's a lot of talk about "faculty governance" at colleges and universities—by both the haters, who think professors are out of control and corrupting the youth, and by those who still aspire to a utopian vision of administrator-free institutions. But the real power always lies with the folks who sign paychecks, making faculty governance a bit of a charade, as well as a major source of frustration and burnout for professors. Suddenly remembering that I was now administration instead of faculty, however, I resolved to say no more and just eat.

"So," Vivian continued, "we wanted to let you know, as a courtesy, that we are planning to bring a resolution to the October faculty meeting, asking for all of our salaries to be made public."

I stopped chewing my last crouton. "Oh?" Vivian had eaten only about half of her salad, pushing the rest around her plate, and Joanne had left all her croutons.

The server came and cleared all the plates except for Barbara's. While still working on her fries, she said, "We have to force the issue now, while we have a new provost and before everyone forgets the trauma of the past year. We just can't let things go back to normal."

"Right," I said.

Barbara continued, "Salary distributions at public universities are more equitable because their salaries are public."

"And the president and last two provosts use confidentiality and 'market forces' as excuses," Vivian continued, "which ultimately benefits the male faculty. We know this because we can see it in the *Chronicle of Higher Education*." The *Chronicle* published salary averages of the nation's colleges and universities every year, which made it clear that all four of them, and several other women, were earning well below the average for their ranks.

"And don't even get me started on the women staff salaries," Barbara added before slurping up the last of her milkshake. *I like her. She has no fucks left to give.*

I listened and nodded and made eye contact.

"So we're really hoping you'll support us," Vivian concluded.

I was considering an appropriate response—one that signaled solidarity without throwing my new boss under the bus before I'd even had a chance to talk with him—when suddenly Joanne excused herself and ran to the bathroom.

"Oh my god," said Elaine, looking down at Joanne's vacated seat. There was a pool of what looked like bright red paint on the vinyl bench cushion. I gasped. The two sitting across the table craned their necks to see. I asked Vivian for some napkins from the rack by the wall and used them to keep the blood from trickling down into the seat crack till we could get a server's attention.

"Is she ok?" I asked.

"Oh, yes," Vivian said, waving her hand and sounding bored, "she's just going through the change. She periodically floods out of the blue like that. I keep telling her it's time for a hysterectomy." She rolled her eyes. "It is simply *life changing* never to have to worry about menstruation anymore!" She pronounced it "men-stroo-ation."

"Well, she's wise to put it off as long as possible," said Elaine defensively. "Those hormone-replacement therapies are dangerous, especially if you have a family history of cancer like Joanne does."

"Then fine, just don't take the hormones!" Vivian preached. "Get osteoporosis and break a hip when you're older!"

"Plus, without a uterus, your innards start falling out your vagina," Barbara added, eating her last fry, her appetite apparently unaffected by the happenings.

This luncheon had taken a weird turn.

"So do some Kegels! It's still better than wearing maxi pads 24/7 and never knowing when you're going to overflow in public." Vivian shook her head. "She said she has to wear two *super plus* tampons and *still* has to change them every *ten minutes* sometimes."

I had successfully stopped the blood from spreading on the fake leather bench but now I didn't know what to do with my hands. We finally succeeded in waving down the server and asked for a wet rag and some more napkins.

"That used to happen to my mom," said Barbara. "I got really lucky—mine just went away one day. I never even got hot flashes."

"You are so lucky," said Elaine. "Did you know perimenopause can last up to a decade?" *A decade?* "For years I used to get my period every two or three weeks, and I had cramps like I was twelve again. And my mom was dead so I couldn't even ask her about it. I was so happy when it finally stopped."

I was starting to feel invisible, for which I was grateful. I decided not to join in. When the server showed up with some wet rags, I thanked her too profusely and together we cleaned up the mess.

Then three phones all dinged at once and they all started reading. It was Joanne, group-texting from the ladies' room. Vivian said, "She's going to sneak out the back door and go home to change. We'll give you a ride back to campus."

I excused myself to go wash my hands. While in the bathroom that Joanne had just vacated, I also used paper towels to dry under my arms and boobs. I had first started sweating in the early months of Covid, and I thought it was just stress. But now I had the creeping sense that maybe it was perimenopause. *Duh, Jen, how have you never had this thought?* And how had my mother never mentioned it? I made a mental note to do some research later.

Joanne had left a drop of blood on the floor next to the toilet. I wiped it up with my damp paper towel. I felt sorry for her, never knowing when her body would betray her in public. It was bad enough we all had to go through the anxiety of getting our periods in the first place as girls, but then as women we also have to go through the whole thing again in reverse. It seemed unfair.

When I went back to the table, the check was still sitting there and I surmised they were waiting for the boss to pay it. Then I realized I didn't yet have an office credit card, so I paid the bill with my personal one. On the ride back to campus, they said they ate lunch together at the diner every Thursday and hoped I would join them again. I thanked them and walked back into the office in a pensive mood. Fran was right where I'd left her.

"I'm back," I said unnecessarily, which elicited another eye-contact-less "Uh-huh." I paused in front of her desk.

"Have you taken a lunch break, Fran?" I asked.

"No, I usually don't," she said, still looking at her computer. "Someone has to stay in the office in case a student comes by."

"Really?" I said, looking out into the empty hallway. Students weren't even back on campus yet. "Even in summer?" She looked up at me then.

"I don't know," she shrugged, "I just follow directions, and this is how we've always done it." Her hand never let go of the mouse. *It's her comfort animal.*

"Well that seems..." I was going to say "stupid" but thought better of it. Maybe there were things I didn't know about why it was this way, although I was pretty sure it was illegal not to give hourly employees a lunch break. "That seems like something we should discuss at our next staff meeting. Maybe we could just, I don't know, put a note on the door that says we're closed from noon to one or whatever. Everyone deserves breaks." She said nothing so I added magnanimously, "Feel free to take one now if you want."

She raised her eyebrows and looked at me briefly before looking back down at the screen. "It's fine."

Chapter 5

Hi, Neighbor

I spent the afternoon trying to set up my calendar for the semester (so many meetings already!), while intermittently answering emails, greeting people who stopped by the office to introduce themselves, and frantically studying the college website to try to learn the names and departments of my new colleagues. I wished someone would just make me a syllabus. (The last guy had left in such a hurry that we'd had no chance for him to help get me up to speed.) Fran left precisely at five and my relief was palpable. I locked the door to the main office, turned out the lights, texted my kids, and worked for another hour or so without interruptions.

When I left, the sun still seemed impossibly high in the sky—a quirk of being on the northwestern edge of the Eastern time zone. The campus was quiet except for a few people passing by with their dogs or taking an evening bike ride. I passed the statue of St. Margaret, casting a long shadow across the lawn. *You died young but least you never bled all over a diner bench.*

At home, Fiona greeted me at the door after spotting me from her windowsill perch. Having a cat was still a new experience, and I realized how much I had missed being greeted at the door by anyone in recent years. I felt winded and exhausted and went straight upstairs to put on comfortable clothes. Kelsey's door was open. She was lying on her bed, her moving boxes apparently untouched. I waved to her and she let out a little scream.

"You scared me!" Her kitty-ear headphones had masked my approach.

"Sorry, hon! I wasn't trying to sneak up on you. I just wanted to let you know I'm home."

"Oh my god, ok, hi." Annoyed, she went back to her phone. *A taste of what is to come.* I sighed. Since I was already annoying my kids, I figured I'd knock on Eliot's door. I wasn't sure if he'd heard but then the door swung open violently.

"What?"

I was surprised all over again at how far up I had to lift my head in order to look him in the eye.

"Hey, bud, I'm home."

"Ok." He let out his breath as if he'd been holding it.

"How was your day?"

"Fine."

"What'd you do?"

"Nothing. Just stuff."

"Ok, well, have you eaten?" This was becoming an interrogation against my best intentions.

"No."

"Are you hungry?"

"I guess."

"I'm gonna change and then I'll see about dinner. Maybe come down around seven?" I was loath to tell him what to do so even my suggestions came out as questions.

"Ok." He closed the door firmly.

I put on a t-shirt and pajama pants and made spaghetti with sauce from a jar. Moose, for all his flaws, was a great cook and would have made it from scratch. I had neither the energy nor the properly stocked pantry for such an undertaking.

Eliot took his bowl back up to his room, but Kelsey and I ate together in front of an episode of *Gilmore Girls*. We remarked on how those crazy girls were forever ordering mountains of food at Luke's diner and then leaving without ever touching it or paying for it. Kelsey gave me the rundown on what her New Jersey friends were doing. Then she added, almost as an afterthought, that she had talked to her father. For some reason that came like a punch in the chest.

"Did you call him or did he call you?"

"He FaceTimed me."

I tried to recover. *You're a grown-up, Jen. He's her father. This is a good thing.* I felt myself growing hotter.

"How's he doing?" I hoped that sounded casual. I tried to slow my breathing.

"Great," she said without enthusiasm. "He's like, 'Look at this sunset!' and 'It's so amazing here, you have to come visit!'" She tried to roll her eyes but I could tell she was fighting tears. "How could he just leave us like that?"

"I know, sweetie." I wanted to hug her but I felt like a furnace, so instead I put my hand on her shoulder and squeezed. "I mean I don't know." *Because it turns out he's just a stupid man-child.* "He's...obviously going through something. Sometimes it happens when men hit middle age. The call it a 'midlife crisis.' But it's not your fault. At all. Not even a little bit, ok?"

"I know." She leaned on me for approximately one second before recoiling. "Ugh, Mom, gross, you're all hot and sweaty!"

I got into my big empty bed that night and turned out the light. I desperately wanted to sleep, but my mind felt like one of those nano bugs trapped in a box, frantically buzzing its way from one wall to the next, finding nowhere to stop and rest. I felt fury at Moose for abandoning our children to go live his best life. I felt fury at myself for getting old, right when they needed a mother with extra energy, and for taking on a new job when I could have kept doing my old job with one hand tied behind my back. Inexplicably, I felt fury at my new house for smelling weird, like dust and old man's hair cream.

A could feel a big, ugly sob trying to break its way up from inside me, but for some reason it never came. It just sat on my chest like an anvil.

When I woke up the next morning I headed to my closet where last night's Jen had remembered to hang up a pant-suit and blouse: a practical uniform for a new administrator. They were a little wrinkled and I was considering ironing them when I heard Kelsey screaming from downstairs. *She's gotten her period!* I thought at first. Then I remembered she'd already been getting it for almost a year. I went to the stop of the stairs and shouted, as calmly as I could, "What'd you say, sweetie?"

"Fiona got outside!"

Shit. Fiona had all her claws but she was meant to be an indoor-only cat.

Until very recently she'd lived under our back porch in New Jersey, where she was born last spring, and Kelsey had wooed her with treats till she would eat right out of her hand. Moose was allergic to cats so there was no possibility of adopting her for real. But in the week after he left and before we moved, Kelsey asked if we could keep her and I didn't have the heart to say no. It was then that Eliot informed me that outdoor cats were an unmitigated environmental disaster, so we brought her inside and bought a litter box. It all happened so fast that I hadn't even taken her to a vet. I made a mental note to find a local one as soon as possible. I didn't want Fiona coming home pregnant and turning her hysterectomy into a kitty abortion, which I would then have to explain to my soft-hearted, already-grieving daughter.

Now the cat was outside. I hadn't showered yet and was still wearing my soaked t-shirt and lounge pants. My saggy boobs were hanging free so I looked around the room for something to cover myself up. I threw on a puffer vest and zipped it, slipping into my flip-flops as I headed out the door.

The sun was already up and it was going to be another hot day. I paused on the porch to look around for Fiona and didn't have to look far. She was right across the street in front of a modest but well-loved mint green house with a rainbow flag and a trans pride flag hanging on either side of the front door. In the yard stood an extremely tall blond in an elegant green shift dress and silver clogs, holding the leash of a small dog. Fiona crouched on top of a birdbath, hissing as the dog barked aggressively at her.

I checked both ways and ran across the street shouting, "Sorry! Sorry! Sorry!"

Just as I got there I tripped on the curb where a tree root had pushed it up a few inches. I felt myself flying forward in what seemed like slow motion. After an eternity, I landed like a starfish on the ground, my legs on the sidewalk and my body on the grass at the woman's feet.

"Oh my god!" said a low voice. "Are you ok?"

I felt a hand land gently on my arm. "HUSH, Deirdre," she said sharply to the beast, who had now turned her attention from Fiona to the vanquished invader in her yard.

I groaned and pushed myself up onto my knees. "Yeah, I'm ok I think." Trying to laugh I added, "I'm gonna feel that tomorrow, though!"

I never used to be clumsy, but tripping and falling was something I now seemed to do on the semi-regular, and it often left me aching for days. The woman helped me stand up and I looked at my hands. They were grass-stained but thankfully not bloody. My favorite, softest pandemic pants now had a hole in the knee. I was shaken and humiliated and tried not to tear up while still struggling to reorient myself.

"I am so sorry," she said profusely. "I've called the city about that sidewalk multiple times but still haven't seen any action." She watched me as I brushed off my vest and knees. "Are you really ok?"

When I finally looked up at her I saw that her hair was actually a mix of strawberry blond and grey. She had a chiseled jaw, a long nose, appealing laugh lines, and a prominent Adam's apple.

"Yeah," I laughed, recovering. "I'll be fine. I just feel like an idiot." She—he? they?—groaned sympathetically. "I just came over to get my cat," I said.

Fiona was now down on the ground chewing on a tall piece of grass while Deirdre, some kind of potato-shaped terrier-pug-Chihuahua-mutt with a pronounced underbite, sniffed Fiona's butt seriously. I picked the cat up. "I'm Jen, by the way, your new neighbor. TA-DA!" I struck a silly pose with my one free, grassy hand and then extended it to her. She took it unreservedly with a broad smile and a chuckle. Fiona loudly mourned the end of her big adventure. Her claws made scratchy sounds on my puffer vest.

"Jamie," she said warmly.

"Oh!" I exclaimed, "You brought us the doughnuts!"

"Yes!" she smiled. Her eyes were green like her dress. "Did you like them?"

"Oh my god, they were so good. I ate about three in a row." *It was four but whatever. And you only stopped at four because you figured you should save at least two-thirds of the dozen for your hungry children.*

"Oh I know," she said. She had a dimple in her left cheek. "I usually only allow myself to buy one at a time, but since you're newcomers I thought you needed a whole dozen. I get them from this Mennonite bakery out by the highway. I can show you sometime."

"No, please!" I laughed, "As you can see, doughnuts are the LAST thing I need." She just smiled. I felt myself blushing. I shook my head and buried my face in Fiona's neck. *Why are you being so weird?*

She kindly changed the subject. "So you work at the college?"

"Yeah, today's my second day. Or it will be if I actually make it there alive. What about you, do you work here in town?"

"Yes, I have a little bookstore downtown. Come by and see me!"

Kelsey came running over. "Hi!" she said to Jamie with a big smile.

"Hello there! I'm Jamie. What's your name?"

"Kelsey." She shook Jamie's hand and then took the struggling cat from me.

"Nice to meet you, Kelsey. Are you in middle school?"

"Yes, I'm starting eighth grade."

"Nice! It's so much better than seventh grade. I went to St. Judy's Middle School too." Kelsey's eyes grew wide. I suddenly remembered that childhood feeling of shock upon realizing that older people used to be young.

"Ok, well, I really have to go," I felt tongue-tied and didn't really want to leave, "but thanks for...finding our cat and...the doughnuts and...for not making fun of me just now."

"Never," she said conspiratorially. "I'll call the city again today and threaten a lawsuit."

"Haha, ok then," I said backing toward the street.

"Careful!" she said with alarm, reaching toward me.

"Mom!" Kelsey yelled.

I pulled my eyes reluctantly off Jamie and turned around to where I had almost fallen off the curb. *Pull it together, Jen.* I made it home and now I was running late. After quickly showering and dressing (wet hair and wrinkled clothing would have to do), I headed for the stairs but noticed Eliot's door was slightly open. I knocked.

A man's deep basso voice said, "Come in." I was surprised to find him up and sitting at his desk.

"Hi, sweetie," I said as non-offensively as I could. "You're up early. Is everything ok?"

"Yeah, well, people were screaming," he said without looking at me.

"Fiona got out but we caught her."

"Ok."

"How's the unpacking going?" He had his computer set up, but as far as I could tell that was the extent of it.

"Fine."

"I'm off to work." He was already done with me. "I met Jamie, by the way. The neighbor who brought over the doughnuts?" No response. "You didn't mention she was trans."

"Whatever." Frowning, he finally looked up at me. "So what?"

"Nothing!" I protested. "It's just, it's kind of an interesting detail, that's all. I had been picturing some old grandma-type person."

"Well, I guess you should stop making assumptions about people."

Chapter 6

Putting on My Big-Girl Pants

I arrived for my second day at the office at 8:03 a.m., slightly less anxious than I had felt yesterday but still sweating. Fran was already there and on the phone. She looked up and gave me a half-hearted wave in response to my overly enthusiastic silent greeting. (Eliot hates the way I compulsively wave at neighbors or even strangers. It's especially bad when I'm in short sleeves and he notices my upper arms flapping half a beat behind my hand.)

I went into my office and closed the door most of the way, leaving it open just a little in case that was the culture here. I turned on the desk lamp, put down my briefcase, and shook out my sore right elbow. I had carried a backpack all through grad school, but when I became a faculty member I had bought myself a beautiful leather briefcase in order to look and feel more sophisticated. I loved it, and it had been alright for a number of years, but as I got older parts of me were starting to hurt. I made a mental note to switch arms now and then on my walk to work.

I turned on my computer and sat down, sipping the coffee I had brought from home while it woke up. I had already dealt with or deleted as many emails as I could from my phone while lying awake at 3:00 a.m., as usual, but there were still 23 unread ones. I skimmed through them. One was from the chair of the board's academic affairs committee, saying she was looking forward to meeting me in October. One was from an anthropology professor (actually *the* anthropology professor) about something to do with Native American artifacts that needed to be returned to their tribe, per a law called NAGPRA that the college had been ignoring since 1990. One was from the Title IX coordinator/diversity and inclusion director hoping to find a date for faculty sensitivity training as soon as possible. And one was from President Festerling, reminding me that my presentation to the cabinet about this year's vision for the academic sector was first on the agenda at our 8:30 meeting today.

Reminding? Today?

My insides turned to jelly and my sweat turned cold. It was 8:06. I searched through my in-box for his previous emails to see if I could find out any more about his expectations. I needed a toilet immediately so I walked as quickly as I could, without running, to the all-gender one-seater down the hall. I just barely sat down before it was too late. While sitting there, I scrolled through my phone and found the email he'd sent last week, asking me to make a presentation about the academic sector at today's meeting. Apparently I had agreed to this and promptly forgotten all about it.

How could I let this happen? Was I really going to start my brand-new job as a sweaty, absent-minded divorcée who was literally losing her shit?

I cleaned myself up with the brown institutional paper towels on the wall, wishing I'd grabbed my purse with the baby wipes I always carried, ever since my digestive and endocrine systems had become so unpredictable. I washed my hands, wiped the sweat off my face, along with the mascara that was already spreading around my eyes, and tried to walk with dignity back to my office. Thankfully Fran had nothing to say to me. I closed the door all the way.

I took a few deep breaths. *You are a professional. You've spoken off the cuff lots of times. This doesn't have to be any different.*

One thing I've learned from decades in academia is that most academics love to hear themselves talk. And talk and talk. This means meetings are always much longer and more annoying than they need to be, so most audiences are grateful when someone delivers a short, well-organized presentation without too many topics or take-aways. It was now 8:14. The conference room was a two-minute walk away, so I had fourteen minutes to come up with something, assuming my bowels didn't demand any more attention. *I can do this.*

At 8:29 I walked as confidently as I could into the conference room. President Norm Festerling was standing near the door and greeted me with a formal handshake. He was younger than I, probably in his early 40s, with intense blue eyes, broad shoulders, stiff posture, and a frozen expression that was hard to read. Several people were sitting at the table, looking at their devices. He asked if I would be needing the projector and I said no. I walked around the table to an empty chair.

Everyone was unmasked so I took my mask off, smiled, and said hello to the people on either side of me, hoping for the best. On my right was the Title IX coordinator/diversity and inclusion director, the only person of color and the youngest person at the table. I thanked her for her email and promised to get back to her today. To my left was the Athletic Director and football coach, a tall building of a man, late Boomer with a mullet, wearing a blue St. Margaret's polo shirt with a gold dragon logo. He gave me a silent nod without unfolding his giant arms. I desperately wanted to take off my jacket but my sweaty blouse made it out of the question.

"Welcome everyone," the president said, "let's get started." Almost everyone looked up from their phones. Still standing, he said, "As you know, today is a special day because we're welcoming our new provost to campus," then gesturing toward me, "Doctor Jennifer Smith-Miglione."

He pronounced it with a hard G and silent E, one of Moose's pet peeves, but I decided to just go with it for now. (I had once been thrilled to change my name from the most boring possible 1970s configuration—Jennifer Lynn Smith—to something with Italian flair, but now it irked. I couldn't decide whether or not to drop Moose's name, which was also my children's name.)

"Jennifer has just arrived from New Jersey, where she was Professor of Italian and Dean of Arts and Sciences at Madison College." I smiled around the table at the bland faces of bored people, except for one older guy with a fuzzy mustache who made a silent "Ooooo" and nodded approvingly.

The president continued, "Welcome, Jennifer, to the College of St. Margaret. Grateful that you're able to join us. Look forward to hearing from you this morning about your vision for the academic sector."

He gestured toward the front of the room and clapped imperceptibly as he sat down, letting me know it was my turn to talk. A few people also clapped politely. I had hoped he would have them all introduce themselves so I could have another minute to compose myself, but it was not to be. I smiled again as I stood up and went to the head of the table, stopping in front of the projector screen. The light shone into my eyes and I held my hand up.

"I won't be needing the projector, actually," I said with a nervous laugh.

Someone turned it off.

"Thanks, everyone," I said, "I'm very glad to be here and I'm looking forward to getting to know all of you." Nervous laugh. "Please call me Jen," I said. "If you call me Jennifer I'll think I'm in trouble!" Another nervous laugh. *God you're such a dork! Quit it!* I was on the verge of hyper-ventilating so I pushed my breath out all the way and held it for a second.

"Are you ok?" a kindly-looking older woman to my left asked quietly. (If I recalled correctly, her title was something like Special Assistant to the President, which probably meant she did all the most annoying parts of his job that his secretary didn't do.) My face must have been beet red. I hadn't really had a chance to cool down since walking to the office. I kept my arms close to my sides and pressed my fingertips together in order to keep from fanning my face.

"Oh yes, fine," I whispered, trying to sound casual. "Just a bit of first day jitters."

I cleared my throat and scanned my brain for the three bullet points I had pulled together not even half an hour ago: *collaboration, communication, compassion.* Sets of three are easy to remember, especially if there's also alliteration involved, and they're also easy for audiences to digest. I talked generically about how we were all here for the same reason—to educate students—so collaboration within and across sectors was crucial to developing shared institutional vision. Then I said proactive, transparent communication was key to our effective collaboration, so we weren't all inventing our own wheels or working at cross purposes.

By then mustache guy (VP for HR, maybe?) had closed his eyes.

Finally, I said compassion was called for because we've all been through a very difficult period of slowly unfolding trauma, so we couldn't expect anyone to bounce back immediately—not the students, not the faculty, and not even ourselves. The Athletic Director rolled his eyes at that; the president looked down at his carefully manicured nails.

Basically, I presented a vision of a vision, rather than a vision *per se.* It was admittedly kind of a bullshit presentation, the best I could do on short notice. But even if I had prepared for weeks, it would have been ridiculous for me to come in on my first day and give them a fully formed vision before I even knew their names, much less their problems. I thanked them again and sat down. The whole thing had taken about five minutes and was followed by more polite applause. I spent the next few minutes trying to cool down and steady my breath.

The Athletic Director assured us that everything was back to normal this year and fall sports would run as usual. The VP for Admissions, a millennial woman, tried to sound positive while talking about our extra-small crop of incoming first-year students, but she also worried out loud about retention and "melt" between now and mid-September. The VP for Advancement (academia's fancy name for fundraising), another Boomer, talked about the large gifts that were rolling in for the new men's and women's e-sports teams as well as the chapel renovation. He also had a seven-figure pledge to endow a brand-new MBA program, if only —he looked right at me—the faculty would approve it. He warned that the general fund had been lagging during the pandemic, but he was sure that would turn around now that things were "back to normal."

The CFO, a white male Boomer (*let's just call them WMBs*), then gave a slide presentation of three possible scenarios for the college's next four years, depending on incoming first-year class sizes. All three scenarios required significant budget cuts due to health care costs, shrinking donations, and high tuition discounts. This then segued into the COO (yet another WMB) excitedly talking about outsourcing to save money. They had already outsourced dining services, housekeeping, and groundskeeping to out-of-state corporations, and now they were working on outsourcing payroll, career services, IT, and mental health counseling. "The opportunities for cost savings are amazing," he beamed. The president nodded approvingly. I raised my hand tentatively.

"I'm sorry I don't know the answer to this already," I began apologetically, "but what's going on with the endowment?" Raising my hand had caused my sweaty underarm hair to itch so I tried to scratch it unobtrusively.

"Oh it's tremendous," said the COO. "The stock market has come way back up in the past year."

"And are we able to cover some of the budget shortfall that way?" I asked.

The COO gave a non-committal "Ummm" and looked at the president.

"Yes, it certainly is becoming a tremendous year for the endowment," Norm said, "and we are grateful that we have this cushion to fall back on in case of emergencies." He cleared his throat. "Of course, we don't want to spend it down unless we absolutely have to, so getting the budget under control is our first plan of attack."

It seemed to me that a never-ending deadly pandemic should count as an emergency, but I decided to keep my mouth shut till I knew more. I made a mental note to ask the president about it at our post-meeting meeting.

It turned out I needn't have bothered because he brought it up preemptively, before my growing butt even landed on his petite office couch.

"Yes, the board is adamant," Norm said, shutting the door, "that we need to trim our budget before they'll consider increasing our draw-down on the endowment. They see the pandemic as an important opportunity for a reset."

Because of course they do.

"Higher ed was definitely due for a reset," I confirmed, trying to establish some agreement. *Don't say 'but.'* "It's also true that board members often favor the blunt instrument of budget cuts, even when more nuanced or mission-driven solutions might be called for." Board members almost everywhere tended to be alumni/ae and big donors who could afford to make large gifts. This meant they overwhelmingly came from the business world, so they sometimes had trouble understanding the myriad ways in which nonprofit institutions were purposefully different than corporations.

"Yes, our board members are very engaged and very generous," he said evenly. "So how are you settling in?" I guessed we were done with that topic. *Stay in your lane.*

"We've still got some work to do but we're getting there. I'm..." I didn't want to say too much, but I thought my boss needed to know, "I'm single parenting now. My husband decided not to move to Michigan with us." True enough and appropriately bland.

"I'm sorry to hear that." Equally bland.

"Thanks. We'll be ok." The tiniest brown bird was checking out the bark of the tree beyond his window.

"Of course."

"Is that your family?" I pointed to a professionally-taken photograph on the wall. A smiling young red-haired woman sat holding a pale infant in tiny overalls. She was flanked by three smiling red-haired girls with their little white hands on her shoulders. They were all wearing matching green velvet and looked like a poster for St. Patrick's Day, or maybe Future Ginger Leaders of America.

"Oh yes, that was a Father's Day gift a few years ago."

"Lovely. How old are they now?"

"Nine, seven, five, and three," he said. *Perfectly spaced out, of course.* "Lots of fun."

"I remember." Like an old person I added, "Enjoy it while you can!"

"Indeed. Well I'm sure you have plenty to do so I won't keep you," he stood up quickly, "but let's plan on meeting again in a week or so after you've settled in. Our assistants can work to arrange a good time."

"Great."

We shook hands and wished each other a good day. I checked the time as I walked back to my office. Only 10:00 a.m. and already I needed lunch and a nap.

What happened to me? I used to work fourteen-hour days without stopping, even to eat, and I felt exhilarated. Now all I could think about was making it to the bathroom and the feeling that I was starving. I made a mental note to buy some snacks to hide in my office drawer.

When I arrived, Fran had messages for me from three different science faculty members who wanted me to go have a tour of their labs and see why their department needed additional funds more than any other department. I didn't think building improvements were part of my job but I would need to find out. While she was explaining these messages to me the phone rang again. Fran answered, listened for a minute, and put her on hold.

"You're gonna want to take this one."

The caller turned out to be my first irate parent, calling to say it was my fault her son had flunked three out of his four classes last semester (everything except athletic training for one credit), and threatening to sue me personally if the college didn't refund the past semester and take him off the probation list in time for the fall football season. I assured her I'd look into it immediately.

All in all, my second morning at the office hadn't been a total disaster, but I wasn't sure how I was going to keep up with all the things now in my column. I hoped this flurry of issues was a matter of pent-up demand, rather than business as usual.

Chapter 7

Pool Party

On the last Saturday in September, I determined to spend at least half of the day unpacking. I still hadn't dealt with all my boxes, which was very unlike me—I was usually pretty good about staying on top of things. I figured unpacking could also count as exercise, which I hadn't had much of lately. After only a few minutes I was sweating profusely so I turned on a fan. Our central air conditioning didn't work very well upstairs, and we were having a string of hot days after a couple of cold ones, the kind of weather people used to call "Indian summer" before we realized it was racist.

Thinking about that reminded me about the Native American artifacts we still had in an archive somewhere that needed to be given back to the local tribes. I thought the anthropologist had told me in an email that we were on Potawatomie and Ojibwe lands (St. Margaret's didn't have a land acknowledgement) but I couldn't remember so I picked up my phone to check. All thoughts of artifacts were forgotten, however, when I saw a text from Jamie and my heart did a little jump.

<Hi, Jen! Swim this afternoon? Kids too!> I loved that she had included a traditional greeting and punctuation in her text, complete with exclamation points.

Apart from my body not being "swimsuit ready," a dip in the pool sounded unbelievably appealing. I walked across the hall to Kelsey's room and found her lying on her stomach across her bed, looking at last year's yearbook. I stopped in the doorway for a moment. She probably missed home, despite already having new friends, and despite being in constant touch with her old friends via SnapChat and Instagram. Or perhaps it was *because* she was in constant touch with her old friends.

"Hey, hon," I said loudly, waving to get her attention. She looked up and lifted one headphone. "Feeling homesick?"

"Kinda," she said. "Bella and Sophia are down the shore today." Bella's parents had a house near the shore in Belmar, to which Kelsey and Sophia had often been invited in the past. "It looks fun." She held up her phone to show me two smiling teenagers making duck lips and peace signs in bikinis on a beach. I felt punched in the chest with envy and sadness on my daughter's behalf. *Shake it off, Jen, you're the mom.*

"Well guess what," I said to interrupt my thoughts as much as hers. "Jamie invited us for a swim today. Wanna go?"

"Right now?" Her eyes grew wide, intrigued.

"This afternoon sometime."

"Awesome!" Kelsey always being up for anything was a thing I would miss terribly once she, like her elder brother, figured out how lame her mother was.

"Do you know where your bathing suit is?" I asked. "I'm still looking for mine."

"I think so." She bounced off the bed and headed for her dresser. Then suddenly her face fell.

"What is it?"

"Um," she hesitated, "What if I get my period?"

"What do you mean?"

"I saw this video that said it's bad to go swimming during your period."

"What?" I asked, incredulous. Is this what they taught girls in Midwestern schools?

She picked up her phone and pulled up a TikTok video, excerpted from some ancient health class movie. A teenage girl in black and white answered an old-fashioned phone in the front hall of a suburban house. Soon after she asked her mother if she could go swimming. Her mother answered something to the effect of, "No, dear, it's dangerous to go swimming during the first few days of your period. You might catch cold." My mouth fell open but I was too stunned to laugh. When the girl said into the phone, "Of course I can't go swimming, you know I have the curse!" I finally let out a guffaw.

"Sweetie," I said, as respectfully as I could, "this video is really old and...inaccurate. It's perfectly safe to go swimming during your period." And because it seemed the right thing to do I hugged her and added, "And it's not a curse!" She seemed relieved and excited and pulled a bikini out of her drawer.

Then I turned and looked at Eliot's closed door. I checked the time and decided to text him instead of knocking. I was constantly afraid of waking him up or—worse—interrupting masturbation (which, based on the lunchroom conversations I recalled between my male friends back in the 1980s, high school boys did nearly constantly). The very best-case scenario was that he was already awake and simply unhappy to see me, crushing my mood and even my self-esteem. I would wait to talk to him till he emerged on his own.

I texted Jamie back. <That would be great! At least Kelsey and I will join you. What time?>

She said 3 p.m., when the sun would be over the backyard. I went back to work with renewed vigor, knowing I had something fun to look forward to. Eventually I located my "mom suit," a one-piece with an attached skirt. *Blerg,* I thought, *now I have to shave.*

The next box I opened contained a couple of books I'd read a few years ago when I had started to feel somewhat disconnected from Moose, who had stopped showing much interest in us spending any quality time together. Even before the pandemic, life had become a mix of work, kids, parents/in-laws, and housekeeping, with nary a date night (much less a weekend getaway or actual vacation) to break up the sameness of it all. With one hand I picked up *How to Fix Your Marriage without Talking about It.* Basically, train your spouse like a pet. With the other, I pulled out *Seven Principles for Making Marriage Work,* written by the purported "country's foremost relationship expert." I hadn't gotten past the first part on "love maps."

I had always heard that parents of teenagers were the unhappiest of married people, so I'd figured Moose and I could ride out these hard years and deal with the fallout later, after the kids were gone. Kind of a late-in-life marital do-over. A second act. Obviously that strategy hadn't worked as well as I'd hoped; I probably should have checked in with Moose at some point to make sure we were on the same page.

My heart started racing and I impulsively threw the books across the room. One hit the wall with a loud crack and bounced back with a thud, while the other flew out the door and slid down the hallway. Fiona, who had been vigorously licking her butt with one hind leg pointed straight up in the air, fled under the bed. I froze, wondering if one of my kids would come running, but no one came. I got down on my knees and looked under the bed.

"Sorry, Fee, won't happen again." I picked up both books and threw them in a big black trash bag.

※

Three o'clock finally rolled around. My room was looking much better and I was exhausted and ready for a break. Eliot, whom I still had not laid eyes on, texted <no thanks> in response to my texted invitation to Jamie's.

Loser, I thought, *but at least he said thanks.*

Kelsey and I put on our swimsuits, sprayed each other on the porch with sunscreen, and flip-flopped across the street. I wanted to bring Jamie something small as a hostess gift but didn't have anything appropriate in the house, so I made a mental note to pick something up next time I was out running errands. I hadn't been to her house before so this was a chance to learn a little bit more about her tastes.

When we arrived Jamie was pulling leaves out of the pool with a net on a long stick. She had large white sunglasses on and a one-piece bathing suit with skinny straps and long sequined fringe hanging down in a kind of rainbow ombré—red at the neckline, orange and yellow at her midriff, green and blue at the bottom. Her toenails were painted to match—red on the big toes, blue on the pinkies.

"Hello, ladies," she waved happily as we let ourselves through the gate, being careful not to let Deirdre escape. I reached down to pat the weird little creature as she sniffed around our feet and was rewarded with wet dog hair stuck to my hand. Deirdre was apparently an enthusiastic swimmer.

Kelsey dropped her towel, kicked off her flip flops, and cannonballed into the pool. As soon as her head resurfaced, Deirdre barked and jumped in after her. I walked around the pool to where Jamie was.

"Do you need any help?" I asked.

"Sure, if you get those last couple of leaves I'll go get us something to drink."

I did as I was told and then slipped off my muumuu and got quickly into the water while she was still inside, so as to avoid the anxiety of undressing in front of someone new. I left my towel strategically beside the stairs for when I got out. The water felt so good. A little cold, but in a way that made me notice how stressed I had been, how tightly I'd been holding myself together. I paddled out to the deep end and dared to let myself float.

She came back out a few minutes later carrying a clear acrylic tray loaded with treats. I was still enjoying the water and wasn't ready to get out. Kelsey got out and grabbed a handful of cherries while Jamie looked on with an absent-minded smile and her hands on her hips. After chewing for a few seconds Kelsey asked, "What should I do with the pits?"

"There's a bowl right here for them, darling," Jamie said, pointing out a little crystal bowl. "Or, if you really want to have fun, we can have a contest to see who can spit them farther." That idea delighted Kelsey, and the two of them spent the next few minutes taking turns trying to blow pits over the back fence, laughing hard and comparing techniques for maximum distance. Deirdre sniffed around the grass at the base of the fence, her tiny tail poking straight up in the air. I got out and wrapped my towel around my hips while they were distracted.

On the tray were three tall glasses of ice, each with a metal straw, and a pitcher of water with cucumber slices and stalks of mint floating among the ice cubes. The Michigan cherries were obscenely red, with an appealing sheen of condensation on their refrigerated skins. I popped one into my mouth and rolled it around on my tongue while I poured three glasses of water. I sorted out the pit with my teeth and put it in the bowl, which seemed way too fancy for collecting garbage that had been in our mouths. Then again, the hostess was currently kicking ass at spitting projectiles into the neighbor's yard.

I plopped down on a chaise, took a sip of cucumber water, and closed my eyes, enjoying the prickly hot feeling of the sun's cancer-causing rays on my chilled, pasty skin. I suddenly had an image of Moose, his Italian skin baked bronze in the Costa Rican sun, walking the beach with his young girlfriend. *Fuck you, pura vida.*

Jamie got a glass and sat down next to me. She said "Cheers" and we clinked glasses. Kelsey took a quick sip of water and dove back into the pool.

"Thank you so much for inviting us over," I said sincerely. "This feels sooo good."

"I'm glad you could come," she said sincerely. "I always wait to close the pool till after the late September heatwave and it's nice to make a party out of it."

"Do you like having a pool?" I asked. "I hear it's a lot of work."

"It is a lot of work," she nodded, "but it's a luxury I really enjoy in the summertime. Most of my vacations are 'staycations'." She made air quotes with her manicured fingers.

I couldn't figure out how to ask a follow-up question that wouldn't seem nosy or rude, so I just said, "Oh?" and hoped that would suffice. It did.

"When my parents were still alive I never liked to go too far away. I'm an only child," she explained, "and they were already well into their 40s when they had me. I grew up just around the corner," she pointed vaguely behind us, "and the people who used to own this house had kids and sometimes let us swim in the pool, which I always loved. So when they retired and moved to Florida I bought it. It was a total disaster. I basically had to gut everything, but now it's perfect for me." She grinned and took a sip of water.

"Have you lived in St. Jutta your whole life then?" I asked.

"Almost," she said. "I was born near Detroit and we moved here when I was a toddler."

"You must know everyone in town then."

"Pretty much," she said. "For better and for worse. My dad was a professor at the college and my mom was an English teacher at the high school."

"Oh!" I was happy to find a connection. "What did your dad teach?"

"Business management," she said with a smirk. She perched her sunglasses on her forehead and looked straight at me. She had on bright blue mascara that made her green eyes sparkle. "So you can guess what he wanted his only son to do with his life."

"Ohhhh," I said, again not wanting to say something stupid. This was the first time she/they had alluded to her/their gender or sexuality and I hoped she/they would keep going. (Honestly, she seemed like a she to me, but I had learned that such things weren't always obvious.)

She pulled her sunglasses back down and leaned her head back on the chair. "Thankfully my mother was more liberal-artsy so she insisted that I do all kinds of impractical things to make me 'well-rounded,'" more air quotes, "like piano lessons and summer arts camps and stuff like that. And then when it came time for me to go to college, my dad wanted me to go to St. Margaret's for free and major in business. He didn't see the point in 'wasting' money on 'useless' stuff."

I loved watching her hands as she talked. They moved elegantly, like a dancer's. She wore a single gold band around her left middle finger, and a stack of mixed metal rings on her right ring finger.

"But my mom encouraged me to apply to Oberlin, where she went. She thought it would be a better fit, and she was right of course."

"So that's where you went?" I asked.

"Yep," she said. "I majored in economics to make my dad happy, but I minored in art history and comparative literature." She took another sip. All the ice had melted. "More importantly, I met a bunch of 'coastal elites' and figured out I was queer."

I made a mental note of "queer." It still didn't answer the question about pronouns.

"Wow, that must have been liberating," I said.

"Oh it was life-changing," she said. "Life-saving, actually. I had spent most of high school in this small town feeling pretty depressed, as you can imagine. And in college I finally found people who got me, you know? Deirdre!" She gasped. "You are taking liberties!"

Deirdre had climbed up onto my chaise and started licking pool water off my ankles.

"She's fine," I laughed, anxious not to lose the thread. "How did your parents react?"

"My mom was wonderful, as always. Of course she had always known. My dad mostly pretended there was 'nothing to see here.' Then after college I moved to Chicago with my girlfriend, which *really* freaked him out because he'd finally gotten used to the idea of having a gay son."

"Oh," I was surprised. "Was it serious?" My bladder was starting to demand attention.

"I thought so at the time, but I was twenty-one so what did I know?" She looked at me and held up her hands like an IDK emoji. "She was my best friend, Heather. It didn't last long. She knew I was queer, of course, but she didn't mind as long as I was monogamous. But I started getting therapy, getting more in touch with myself, yadda yadda yadda, and then I started wearing women's clothes and going to drag shows, and she wasn't up for that." She shrugged. "We were still just stupid kids, really. Anyway, I moved back here about a decade ago to be close to my parents when my mom got dementia."

"Are you still in touch with her? Heather?"

"A little bit, mostly just on social media. We've both moved on but I think we've worked our way to good feelings about each other. At least I have."

"Wow," I said stupidly. My bladder now refused to be ignored. "I'm so sorry to interrupt but could I please use your rest room?"

I followed her directions into the house to the windowless powder room just inside. I switched on the light and struggled out of my wet suit. From my throne, I took in the room, which was painted black from floor to ceiling. My feet rested on a fuzzy silver rug. A cabinet hung above the sink, with small retro light bulbs perched on top. The lights reflected off a dozen tiny disco balls waving from the ceiling on fishing wire, creating tiny specs of light every-where. When I got up I saw tiny words painted on the cabinet mirror and leaned in to read them: "You are per-fect." I couldn't help opening it, and was rewarded with the words "GO ON WITH YOUR BAD SELF," filling the inside of the door. On the shelves were mints, dental floss, some tampons in a silver cup, a stick of SPF 70 sunblock, and a bottle of ibuprofen—a thoughtful collection of things a pool guest might need.

"I love your bathroom!" I announced upon my return. Jamie and Kelsey were both in the deep end, hanging off the side of the pool by their elbows. I sat down next to Kelsey and dangled my feet in the water. Briefly feeling embold-ened by Jamie's mirror messages, I went for it. "Forgive me for asking, Jamie, but before we leave the subject entirely, would you mind telling us your pronouns?"

"Mom!"

"It's fine, darling—I really am confusing, aren't I? I dress like a woman, but I also haven't gone to the trouble of surgically making myself *look* like a woman."

Kelsey and I both waited.

"At some point I just started wearing whatever I wanted, which turned out to be women's clothes most of the time. And then once my hair grew out a little and I started wear-ing eye makeup, some people just started to call me she, and I liked it. It felt right. Although when I go running I'm pretty much still just a dude with a man bun."

We all laughed.

"I mean, I was he for the first half of my life and I still feel connected to that boy and that young man. And I haven't changed my legal documentation so I'm not 'officially' a woman in any way that most people would recognize. In millennial terms I'm 'non-binary,' which fits pretty well, but yeah, 'she' is the way to go." She ended with a decisive nod.

"Would you ever go by 'they'?" Kelsey asked. I was surprised and pleased. *Kids these days, with their tolerance and understanding.*

"Oh no, darling, I'm way too Gen X for that," she waved it off like something that smelled bad. "And frankly too much of a grammar snob!"

"Right?" I laughed. "Old habits die hard. Although apparently the singular 'they' goes way back."

"Ugh, I know." She shook her head. "Don't get me wrong, I'm totally fine calling *other* people they! It just doesn't work for me. I've used 'queer' for decades and I still like it because for me it covers everything—a gender-fluid, bisexual, trans woman. I just want to be who I am, which is...Jamie!" She threw back her head in a concluding flourish.

I stared at her in awe. She seemed so completely at peace with herself. What must that be like? People who didn't know her might think she was eccentric, and I suppose she kind of was. But she was also perhaps the most down-to-earth person I'd ever met. I couldn't figure out why she would want to hang out with someone so vanilla like me. She was probably just being kind.

"That's so cool," Kelsey said, pushing off and diving back under. Jamie and I went back to our chaises to drink more water and eat more cherries. When we got settled, Jamie pushed her sunglasses up on her head and looked me in the eyes.

"So how about you? How are you holding up? Kelsey told me a little bit about your divorce." I wasn't ready for that.

"Oh, yeah, no, I'm fine, you know?" I managed. She waited. "I mean, it's a lot. A lot of changes all at once." She nodded sympathetically, squinting above her freckled cheekbones. The late afternoon sun and the breeze made her soft-looking hair glow like a halo. I imagined touching it.

"Did you know I met your husband, ex-husband, when he came to buy the house last month?"

"No! Really?" He hadn't mentioned it. Then again, he hadn't mentioned leaving me until the last possible minute.

"Yes, we met on the street," she said. "Except he told me his name was Matt."

"Right," I said, "Matthew Junior. His dad went by Matt so I guess the family needed a different nickname for him." She waited again. "I think it's been really hard on the kids, him leaving right before we moved."

"I would think so. Moving is a lot. And hard on you too. You've all been through so much. *Are going* through so much."

She looked at me so attentively that I felt my eyes tear up. I still hadn't cried even once about Moose leaving and I was afraid I was going to start at this very moment. She had just told me a bunch of her life story, and it seemed right that I should tell her some of mine, but it was still too humiliating, too raw.

"It's really hot," I said, sighing loudly and rubbing my nose hard with my towel. "I think I might jump in again."

I looked toward the pool but made no effort to get up. Kelsey was doing a handstand, her legs pointing straight up out of the water. I could suddenly remember the exact feel of doing underwater handstands in my childhood neighbors' pool, my hands on the scratchy bottom, my shins and feet in the open air while my body wobbled upside down and I blew bubbles into the blue blur to keep the water out of my nose. When was the last time I had done that?

"That's a marvelous idea," Jamie said, kindly looking away.

Kelsey's head reemerged from the pool, her eyes squeezed closed as she inhaled loudly and wiped hair and water out of her face. Jamie laid her sunglasses on the table and shouted, "Ready or not, here I come!" before leaping and making a huge cannonball into the deep end.

Chapter 8

Downtown

As October approached, my little family was easing into something like a "new normal." Or at least that's what everyone kept saying.

We were (mostly) unpacked and feeling more at home in our house. I had helped Kelsey hang posters on the walls and twinkle lights on the ceiling of her bedroom. Eliot had discovered that if he showered late at night, the hot water would last nearly an hour before going cold. I had finally located the carafe to the automatic coffee maker and installed it in a prime spot on the countertop. And I had used magnets to stick a bunch of the kids' school pictures and family photos up on the old refrigerator that came with the house. (Our last fridge had been stainless, so this throwback to my childhood was kind of a novelty.) I had to keep them stuck near the top of the doors, though, lest Fiona have her predatory way with them.

Kelsey had survived the first few weeks at the middle school with relatively little drama, apart from a couple of the boys telling her she stank like an armpit because she came from New Jersey, the armpit of the nation. She was generally a crowd pleaser, neither freakishly beautiful nor pitifully strange looking, not overly self-conscious, quick to laugh, and genuinely curious about other people. She had already been to a slumber party, where half a dozen girls counseled each other about bras and periods and kissing, and tried to one-up each other about who was the most devoted Swiftie. I knew this because she still told me everything.

Kelsey's social life was on fire compared to Eliot's. He went to school and cross country and then came straight home and went up to his room till shower hour. Unlike my tween daughter, my teenage son told me nothing. If I was lucky, he would make a brief appearance for half an hour or so in the evening, when we all sat together and watched an episode of *Community* or *Doctor Who* or some other silly show while we ate dinner. (I had given up on dinners at the table out of self-preservation. I just couldn't handle the full-on scorn from my firstborn right now, even for twenty minutes.) I would try to find out as much as I could about his life in ten-second snippets, during the credits or between scenes here and there. I also tried to toss in whatever occasional life lessons I could glean from the shows we watched, since he had stopped tolerating my sermons long ago, even before his father left.

On a beautiful autumn Sunday, Kelsey consented to wander downtown with me to visit Jamie's bookstore, which we still hadn't seen. She was having her period and was feeling grumpy and crampy. I let her spend most of the day on the couch but convinced her to take a little walk with me that afternoon, plying her with ibuprofen and promising her the fresh air would do her good. I really was becoming my mother.

Every step she took seemed reluctant so—in an effort not to become my mother entirely—I forced myself to slow down rather than hurry her along.

"I can *not* believe I have to get my period every month for like a million years," she said. "I feel so *gross.*"

"I know, sweetness, it does feel gross sometimes," I soothed. "You're *not* gross, but I'm sorry you're feeling bad."

"What if I don't have PMS and this is just my regular personality?"

I laughed and put my arm around her shoulders. "It is *not* your personality. Or at least not your whole personality. You are delightful and energetic and curious and amazing. Everyone gets to have a bad day now and then."

Then I had a thought. "You know, I used to think PMS made me irrational, because there were only a few days a month when I just couldn't seem to put up with things. I would scream at you guys, or cry about the news, or get angry about nonsense at work. When the rest of the month I could usually keep some level of equanimity.

"But now I think maybe it wasn't irrational to sometimes feel rage about stuff. The world really is a stressful place, and life isn't easy. And some days you notice it more than other days, because you're exhausted or your emotions are closer to the surface or whatever." I was babbling. "Anyway, just think, someday you'll be like me and you won't have your period for like...months at a time!" *How many months has it been?* "And someday you'll never get it again!"

"Yeah, but you're *old,*" she whined.

"Hey!" I protested, trying to convince myself. "I'm only 51!" *Almost 52.* "That's not even close to old!"

"But that's like, 37 years away!" I mentally checked her arithmetic. She always did have a good head for numbers. She'd probably become an accountant and start out-earning me right after college.

"You'll make it, I promise. Come on, I'll buy you a fun book and then we can go get some ice cream."

Jamie's bookstore was called Flyover Pride Books. It had a shiny pink and black painted exterior with pride flags in the windows and a hand-wrought iron and wood sign dangling over the door like a British pub. It was as if a bit of Stars Hollow, Connecticut had erupted in the middle of Cicely, Alaska. A sign on the door said, "Mask-Friendly Space," so we pulled ours out and put them on.

A bell jingled as we entered. Familiar voices singing "...and we can treat people with kindness...find a place to feel good" wafted over the little shop, along with the scent of herbal tea. "Welcome in," said a young man in a mask from behind the plexiglass screen at the counter, and we reciprocated.

The display table closest to the door was covered in books by Midwestern authors, from Hemingway and Mary Oliver to Jonathan Franzen and Malcolm X. There were also several travel guides with titles like *Meet Michigan* and *Midwest Road Trip*. I picked up a paperback called *The Lager Queen of Minnesota*, while Kelsey made a beeline to the YA section in back.

She had torn through the Harry Potter books at age nine and quickly moved on to the Percy Jackson series, and then *The Hunger Games*. I hadn't let Eliot read Harry Potter till he was eleven (I figured Harry was eleven in book one so that was the right time) or *The Hunger Games* till he was thirteen (a few years younger than Katniss, but he wanted to see the movies so I made him read the books first). But younger kids want to do whatever their older siblings are doing and they tend to get away with it. After a long vampire phase thanks to *Twilight*, she was now into stand-alone novels in which teen romance figured prominently.

"Kelsey, darling!" said a familiar voice. I looked up from a shelf of books on sobriety to see Jamie emerging from the doorway marked "Fabulous Employees Only, Darling." She hugged my menstruating daughter, who enthusiastically hugged her back. Upon seeing this, a warm feeling filled my chest and I froze for a moment. Then Jamie waved at me, breaking the spell, and I walked toward them.

"Hello, sweetie," she said to me as we hugged. When we parted I let my eyes take her in. She was wearing green wide-leg trousers, pink European-looking sneakers, and a royal blue sweater, above which emerged a lacy white collar with a string of pearls peeking out from underneath it. Above her shiny blue KN-95 her green eyes crinkled in a smile. In an exaggeratedly formal voice she said, "And what brings you ladies in today? Can I help you find something special?"

"Ugh, I have cramps," Kelsey blurted, surprising me, "and Mom made me take a walk for my mental health." I hadn't specifically said these words to her and wondered where she'd gotten them. Not that she was wrong.

"Oh, my poor baby," Jamie said, putting her arm around her shoulders. "We must get you some feel-good literature then. Have you read *Heartstopper* yet?" She grabbed a few books off a nearby shelf and got Kelsey settled into a bean bag.

"I notice you still sell Harry Potter," I said, when she returned. *What the fuck, Jen?*

"Guilty," Jamie said. "They're wonderful books that almost single-handedly got two generations of kids to enjoy reading."

"It's just that, I thought J.K. Rowling got, you know, cancelled."

"Oh, she absolutely did."

"For being transphobic."

"Well, the way I see it, she's just really afraid of men. Her first husband was an abuser and a stalker."

"But didn't she tweet some really obnoxious things and then double down on them later instead of apologizing?" I was suddenly ashamed of how little I actually knew about it. And why was I pushing on a controversial topic with a near-total stranger?

"Yeah," she sighed, deflating, "she is pretty much a total idiot when it comes to trans people. I mean, I want to affirm people who are doing their best to think critically and speak their truth, but she seems to think trans women are basically men who wear disguises so they can go into women's spaces just to hurt women."

"Yikes."

"Yeah. But," she perked up again, "before she was openly an idiot, she wrote some great books that have been really important for at least two generations of queer American misfit kids—including me, even though I read them in my thirties. So I like to pretend Harry Potter emerged *ex nihilo.* Plus," she whispered, leaning in, "I only sell used copies, which means Joanne doesn't get any royalties from them."

She smelled like soap and peppermint.

"That's really generous of you, giving her the benefit of the doubt."

"Meh," she waved, "I try to give people the benefit of the doubt whenever I can. I never know when I might need someone to do the same for me. I generally find it easier to go through life when I'm not angry at every single person who says something offensive."

"Easier said than done," I said.

"It takes a lot of practice, but—I don't know, Jen, you strike me as a pretty even-handed person. I bet you're better at it than you think."

"Maybe." *Come to think of it, a little too even-handed sometimes.* "I should actually probably get a lot angrier than I do. That's what Moose used to say. There's just... so much in the world to be angry about that it's hard to know where to start." Lately I'd been feeling like my inner 1995 Alanis Morisette was threatening to cut herself loose from my belly.

"Amen to that, sister."

After a moment, the shadow of a frown came over her eyes and she threw up her hands. Whispering again, so as not to disturb Kelsey, she said, "I mean, as if *any* jerk can't walk into *any* women's room, with or without a dress on, and assault *any* woman or girl *anytime* he wants!" I marveled watching her wrestle with her frustration. "I just wish she'd stay off Twitter. It does not! lend! itself! to nuance! Joanne!" She said, clapping on each word. Then she sighed loudly and composed herself dramatically, which made me laugh. She laughed too, and shook her head.

I wanted her to keep talking. "How long have you had this bookstore?"

"About three years."

"What were you doing before that, after you came back from Chicago?"

"I worked in HR at Eastern Michigan University. When my parents died they left me everything, and I was sick of all the higher ed bullshit—no offense—and St. Jutta had never had a good bookstore, so..." She held her arms up in a jubilant Y and spun around in a circle.

"It's wonderful," I said sincerely. "Has it been a good move for you?"

"It's had its ups and downs. It's not that easy to start a new small business in an economically-depressed state, in a dying college town, and then in a pandemic, but people here have been really supportive. And I still do a little remote HR consulting on the side, so I can pay for my fashion habit. I'm thinking of opening a consignment shop next door once I've paid off the start-up loan for this one. By then I'll be an experienced *entrepreneuse.*"

I was in awe. I could never imagine having the courage to start a business from scratch.

"Can we go get ice cream?" Kelsey called from across the room. "Also I need help getting up." Jamie and I went to her and pulled her out of the beanbag by her hands. Kelsey had a stack of books including *Why We Broke Up*, *Firekeeper's Daughter*, and the first book in a new fantasy series about a girl who kills a wolf and then is terrorized by a faerie. I also bought a copy of Judy Blume's *Are You There God? It's Me, Margaret.*, just because it seemed relevant to her current situation. I wanted to read it again even if she didn't.

Amid our new normal, there were still a number of things I hadn't done related to the maintenance of our lives. Our little lawn was mowed (a useful skill Moose had given both our children), but the car hadn't had an oil change lately and I hadn't even thought about snow tires. Eliot had a sports physical over the summer back in New Jersey, but Kelsey and I hadn't had checkups in over a year and I hadn't yet looked into finding local doctors for us.

And—most inconvenient when my tooth cracked on a Friday morning—we didn't yet have a local dentist.

<Help!> I texted Jamie. <I desperately need a dentist! [Tooth emoji, grandma emoji]>

We had started texting pretty regularly about random things, and sometimes the best part of my day was hearing the "synth" text tone that I had chosen to signal her attention coming my way.

I looked for something to put my tooth fragment in while waiting for her to reply and settled for a peanut butter jar from the recycling bin.

<Oh no! [Ouch emoji]> Jamie texted back. That she used copious emoji, in addition to punctuation, endeared her to me immeasurably. <Hold on...>

A moment later she sent the link of a local dental practice, Heiderscheidt & Heiderscheidt. <Right downtown. They are great.> A moment later, <Father & daughter team. I used to babysit the daughter.>

<Thank you so much! [Grateful hands, smiley face]>

I immediately called the dentist. A female voice said something so quickly that it took me a moment to process. Eventually my brain translated it into, "Heiderscheidt, Heiderscheidt, and Elenbaas, how may I help you?"

"Hello?" came the voice again when I hadn't responded.

"Yes, hi!" I explained my emergency. It turned out neither of the Doctors Heiderscheidt were available that day, but their brand-new associate, Dr. Elenbaas, could see me that afternoon. I went to work as usual, but spent the whole morning trying to minimize actually talking to anyone face to face, full of anxiety that someone would notice me crumbling apart before their eyes in real time.

When the hour finally came, I told Fran I had "an appointment," and walked the short distance to downtown. It felt good to be moving outdoors. It was one of those glorious autumn days where the sun shines kind of sideways. The breeze made the trees whisper and flicker in a mix of green, orange, red, and yellow. I felt a pang of gratitude in my chest that almost immediately turned to grief at the passing of time. I felt myself about to tear up so I shook it off and slowed my pace a little, in an attempt not to arrive at the dentist sweaty, weeping, and out of breath.

When I got to the address, one block off the main street, I did a double take. The dental practice was in an old train depot. But inside everything was freshly renovated and modern, possibly the nicest dentist's office I'd ever seen. There were a lot of people behind the desk, some in masks, some not. Upon checking in as a new patient, I had to fill out a bunch of forms with questions that seemed irrelevant to my teeth (did they really need to know how little I exercised?).

After a few minutes, a hygienist about my age, wearing a blue lab coat and sporting what could only be called "frosted" hair, called me back.

"Hi, Jennifer, I'm Denise. I hear you have a broken tooth."

"Yep." I handed her the jar, trying to "smize" over my mask.

"Oh dear," she said seriously, taking the jar.

"Yeah, it's like things started falling apart right on cue after I turned 50."

She laughed. "Well you've come to the right place for this, at least."

In the exam room, she had me wash my hands and rinse out my mouth at the sink. I understood why, but it made me feel a bit like an undesirable. Once I was seated, we chit-chatted about the weather and me being new in town, till she put on gloves and had a look in my mouth so she could prepare the dentist for what he would see. In a quiet voice she said, "We're ready for Doctor in room 3." I was confused till I realized she was wearing an inconspicuous headset with a microphone.

When the dentist himself entered the cubicle and introduced himself, I was taken aback. He was tall, blond, and gangly, and the face behind the plexiglass shield looked too young to shave. I dutifully resisted making any Doogie Howser references. He pulled up his mask, leaned way over to have a look in my mouth, and assured me this would be an easy fix.

"I don't know why this happened," I said. "I wasn't even chewing anything at the time."

"It looks like maybe you grind your teeth at night," he said. "Do you ever wake up with a sore jaw?" I admitted that I did. "Have you been under any stress recently?" *Oh, child, you have no idea.* I admitted that I had. "Sometimes that can do it, especially for women your age."

I was startled. "What do you mean?" *You know damn well what he means, Jen.*

"Well, as women get older—not that you're old!" he hastened to add, "—but as women go through menopause, their mouths can get drier, which can gradually lead to more tooth decay if you don't correct for it. Like, sometimes with really elderly women, we find that a procedure that should be fairly straightforward accidentally ends up fracturing their jawbones." I must have looked horrified because he quickly added, "That's never happened in my hands, thankfully."

Probably because this is your first day on the job.

What I said out loud was, "I would have thought just the opposite. Isn't a wet environment more conducive to bacteria?"

"Yeah, you'd think so," he said, "but actually the saliva helps wash the gums, and it contains a lot of the good bacteria that fights the bad bacteria."

The more you know.

He left for a few minutes while the hygienist pulled all the necessary tools together for the procedure.

"The thing I've found about menopause," she said quietly, "is that I'm so moody sometimes! I just feel furious and ready to snap at everyone. My OB/GYN just put me on an antidepressant so we'll see if it helps." I made non-committal but sympathetic sounds. Shaking her head she added, "Not getting a period is the *only* good thing about menopause that I can see."

I was lost in thought about all the things that could go wrong in a post-menopausal body and didn't ask from what other symptoms she might be suffering.

After a successful procedure, I made a follow-up appointment for a thorough cleaning and a fitting for a bite guard to wear at night. I also set up appointments for the kids, thankful that I had opted to buy dental insurance when I started my new job. I left the station-office with my face feeling swollen and numb on one side. It was hard to talk and I couldn't stomach going back to work so I walked straight home.

The kids arrived a few minutes after I did. Kelsey came in and gave me a hug, surprised to see me. I asked her how school was and she said it was "boring but fine" and then danced out of the room. Eliot grunted and made a wide circle around me to go look in the pantry, which reminded me there was very little food in the house that wasn't canned chickpeas. He settled for a bowl of quick oats.

"Sorry, hon," I said, "I'll go to the store tonight." Then to deflect I asked, "No cross country today?"

"It's canceled because of homecoming," he said. "We're supposed to run on our own."

"Oh," I said. "Is that tonight?" My tongue still felt funny and it came out "Izzat tonigh'?"

Eliot frowned. "The football game is tonight. The dance is tomorrow."

He put a bowl of oats and water in the microwave and turned it on, looking regretful to be stuck in the kitchen alone with me for another three minutes. Then he said something I didn't expect. "I have a hot date."

"You..." I stared at him stupidly while my brain caught up with my short-term memory. "What?" *Good job, Jen, real cool.*

"He's going to the homecoming dance tomorrow!" Kelsey filled in helpfully, dancing back into the room. Eliot winced.

"Oh!" I said. "Great!" No more information was forthcoming. "With whom?"

"Someone from cross country."

My brain was on fire, and I could feel the heat taking over my torso. I made a detour.

"Don't you have a meet tomorrow?" It was his first Saturday meet and I was planning on going. I felt guilty because I'd missed all the weekday ones so far, thanks to all my committee meetings. I hadn't planned on being a single mom in my first year as a brand-new boss-who's-not-really-the-boss.

"Yeah," he said, leaning awkwardly against the counter, his backpack still on one shoulder, so he could make a quick getaway. "That's in the morning."

I now felt ready to take on the buried lede and tried to sound nonchalant. "So what's her name? Or his name?"

"Her, and never mind." He was visually disgusted at my attempt to be open-minded, but since he'd never had a date in his life, I really couldn't be sure.

"He won't tell us," Kelsey said with a pout, "he's afraid we'll look her up online." He was right of course—what's social media for if not so mothers can stalk their children? I cursed the fact that I didn't have even a minimal moms' network in St. Jutta that I could go to for answers.

"Did you ask *her?*" I asked.

"She asked me," he said coolly. *Oh my god,* I processed, *someone asked my silent, surly boy to a dance.* Did I detect the slightest hint of swagger?

"Wow!" I said. "I mean, great! That sounds like fun." I paused to see if he would offer up anything else. When he didn't I asked, "Do you need anything? Like, a tie, or flowers, or money for a ticket or whatever?"

"I already took care of all that," he said.

I realized, again with a mix of shock and delight, that this had probably been brewing for a while. I wondered if Moose already knew. Kelsey told me he called them fairly often, which was really the least he could do, but for which I was thankful. He also transferred money into my bank account every two weeks. I knew from friends' horror stories that responsible ex-husbands are not to be taken for granted, especially where kids and money are concerned, so I accepted this as a small mercy.

The microwave hadn't finished beeping when Eliot popped open the door and grabbed the bowl with a towel, spoon already in hand.

"OK then. That sounds great." I was at a loss and now repeating myself. "I hope you have fun."

"OK," he replied, his back to me as he fled the scene.

I stood there, dumb with wonder and amazement. My kid, who pretty much never talked to me anymore except under duress, and then only said snarky things, had somehow made a good enough impression in his first month at a new school that someone thought he would be a good date for a dance. I said a silent prayer thanking this mystery girl for seeing something in my boy, sending her wishes that he would be nicer to her than he was to me.

"Mom," Kelsey said, interrupting my pondering, "do we have anything to eat?"

Chapter 9

Homecoming

Eliot had to be up and out of the house very early on Saturday to catch the team bus to the meet. I would need the car to get there later, so I drove him to the high school in the half light, breaking the silence only to say, "Love you, see you there," as he slouched out of the car.

I went home for an hour to take a shower and eat some breakfast. When I looked in the mirror I saw my dad staring back at me. Once upon a time, I used to have something like a chin that was separate from my neck. But suddenly—or so it seemed to me—there was no dividing line between them. *I'll bet Nora Ephron never felt this bad about her neck.* I held my chin out, turned my head left and right. If I made a concerted effort I could still kind of recreate something like what used to be, but the writing was on the wall. My resting face was well on its way to being chinless. Or multi-chinned, depending on the angle.

I had known this was coming, of course. When Moose and I first fell in love I warned him that I was going to get jowly someday, and it was funny back when I thought we'd get old together. Now I could actually see the promised jowly face in the mirror, threatening to tear up, and I felt my heart start racing. It wasn't funny anymore. My brain fast forwarded to my future face—I saw myself beside my dad, my grandmother, my great aunts—a whole host of elderly humans wearing built-in turtlenecks. (It was the one thing that ever made me feel sorry for Mitch McConnell.) Their face was becoming my face, and it was only going to get worse from here on out.

And now I was alone. Any new partner I might find would never know me when I had a real chin, a young neck. They wouldn't have any memory of someone young and beautiful-ish. They would only have middle-aged me, a rapidly expanding, drooping pile of meat on her way to looking like Jabba the Hutt. I might as well paint myself green already.

I am going to be alone forever, I thought. *Moose left me right when no one will ever want me again.*

"Do I have to go today?" Kelsey stood in the doorway, looking gloriously dewy, even straight from her pillow. *She woke up like this.*

"You don't want to go watch your brother run?"

"Ughhhh, it's so booooooring."

"Are you fine staying home alone?"

"Mom, *yeee-ess-uh*! I'm thirteen!"

I couldn't blame her. Staying in jammies and having the house all to myself sounded pretty good. I briefly worried about safety, but then remembered that we now lived in a small Midwestern town, where the reduced numbers of human beings in our vicinity greatly reduced any parental anxiety I had about some random psychopath attacking my daughter. At least until she went off to college.

I plugged the meet location into my phone. It was more than an hour away, but I had always enjoyed a solitary road trip. I cued up a higher education podcast on the topic of trauma-informed pedagogy, and how it should be applied not only to students but also to faculty—since everyone and their brother was suffering mentally from the last few years of living in the U.S., no matter the particulars of their life situation.

In only a few minutes I was outside of town and driving through farmland. I hadn't really noticed how flat Michigan was, allowing me to see long distances in all directions. *Big sky country*, I thought with delight.

By now the sun was shining from the east, making the fields of green and gold seem to glitter. Red barns, white farmhouses, and silver cylinders popped up here and there as I made a long zig-zag across the state. One field was full of fat yellow hay bales. An ancient-looking weeping willow stood alone on a lawn. Another had some kind of impossibly huge farm machine slowly pulling a giant rake across rows of something. Soy? Sugar beets? (If it wasn't corn I had no idea.) I made a mental note to do some research later. It was still a little chilly out, but I cracked my window to let in a bit of fresh morning air. It smelled of fresh grass and manure. For a few moments I felt so good.

Then, a moment later, I felt sad because I hadn't noticed till just then how long it had been since I'd felt good. *Shake it off, Jen, you don't have time for self-pity.*

Being a cross country parent was one of my favorite things about having a kid in high school. Even in the deep pandemic, when school was online, runners were allowed to run, which was important for Eliot since it was pretty much the only time he left the house.

I absolutely hate running—it feels to me like dying—but I love watching other people run. The first time I noticed this was one midnight back in grad school, when the Princeton sophomores stripped naked and ran around a quad in celebration of the winter's first snow—all genders, all body types, fast and slow, some in caps or mittens or scarves, bouncing and floppy and muscular, shrunken and goosebumped from the cold. It felt magical, like I had stumbled upon a festival meeting of ancient deities. Much later, when I started attending cross country meets, I realized the magic of that evening wasn't predominantly in the runners' nakedness, or even in the snow-lit darkness, but in the running itself. I can hardly fathom it, how they just keep their bodies moving. Some of them almost seem to fly.

The final mile of my drive was down a gravel road. I stopped at the entrance of a hunting club to pay my five dollars and get directions to the parking area—a muddy lawn—from a teenager in a yellow vest. The minivan complained as I drove it slowly over countless ruts and bumps on the way to the end of a row of pickup trucks and SUVs. I hoped I would be able to get out when it was all over.

I walked a couple of minutes through the mud to the starting line, where all the teams had little tents set up. I looked for the red and gold "St. Jutta Saints" banner and headed over, trying to put on my most confident and friendly face since I didn't know a soul. The tent was full of backpacks and hoodies and water bottles but empty of people. Up ahead girls were lining up and stretching, ready to start their race, while the boys were off in the distance somewhere warming up. I always thought it was weird how much running the kids had to do to warm up, only to then run the race, and then do still more running to cool down. I guessed that's how they weeded out the non-runners.

When I neared the starting line I positioned myself near some folks in St. Jutta sweatshirts, hoping for an opening to talk to someone. I took my chance when there was a lull.

"It's a beautiful day for a meet," I said in the direction of a woman with dyed red hair and a red and gold Gryffindor-style scarf on. A good deal younger and thinner than I, she smiled at me politely.

"Yes, it sure is," she replied.

"Do you have a runner in this race?" I asked.

"Yes," she said, "my daughter, Anna. She's a senior at St. Jutta." She nodded toward the team of girls, dressed for summer and hopping up and down in the morning chill.

"Oh," I said, "my son is a senior too. Eliot."

"Oh, you're Eliot's mom!" she exclaimed. "They're going to homecoming together."

Aha! I had gotten lucky in choosing my target. Just then the pop gun went off and the girls started running. The woman, whose name I didn't yet know, shouted "Come on, Saints!" and then ran off with the other spectators to meet the group at the next bend in the three-mile course.

I decided to save my energy for chasing the boys' race so I wandered around aimlessly for the next fifteen minutes, trying not to look at my phone so as to appear approachable. No one approached me. Eventually I ended up at the finish line with the cheering crowd. I hadn't thought to wear boots and my feet were wet and cold in their sneakers. When I looked down I noticed there were little shards of plastic all over the ground, I guessed from some kind of shooting practice. *Plastic is the devil*, said Eliot's voice in my head.

I clapped for the girls as they returned, puffing visible breaths into the air, and then moved back toward the starting line where the boys were lining up. I caught Eliot's eye and dared a small wave, which elicited a barely perceptible nod from him. Despite emerging from my reluctant womb and my slow-ass gene pool (I will absolutely be among the first to get eaten in the apocalypse), Eliot was an excellent runner. This was all thanks to Moose; both of them were slight of frame and wiry of build. When he was little Eliot had wanted to do everything his father did, so he'd started running almost as soon as he started walking. Like baby Forrest Gump.

I took some pictures of the team and then prepared to high-tail it around the course. It had been easier to follow him back in junior high, but as Eliot got faster, the courses got longer, and I got older, it had grown harder and harder to keep up with him. I half envied the moms of the slow kids. Now I generally went straight from the starting line to the finish line, with perhaps one stop in the middle if the course wound close enough for me to get there before him.

In New Jersey, where high schools were huge, Eliot had usually finished in the middle of the pack. But today he came in sixth, the second runner from his team and, I was proud to note, the first short boy to cross the finish line. I just barely had time to catch it on video.

I was feeling magnanimous and texted his time and a picture to Moose, but apparently I was too far out in the boonies for the picture to go through. "Message failed to send." I put my phone back in my pocket to try again later. I could tell Eliot was pleased with himself because he almost smiled when I approached him near the water cooler, and he even let me give him a side hug before going back to cheer on the rest of his slower teammates in their final stretch.

"Eliot did well," someone behind me said. Anna's mom again.

"Yes he did—thanks! He definitely doesn't get it from me," I added with a nervous laugh. "I'm Jen, by the way." I started to extend my hand but then stopped myself, not knowing if she was a hand shaker in Covid times.

"Amy," she said.

"How did Anna do?" I asked. "And which one is she?"

Amy turned and indicated a dark-haired girl in two French braids and a knee brace. "She had a pretty good day," she said, "but she's still recovering from an injury, so not a PR."

"Aw," I said sympathetically. I was spared from having to figure out what to say next. "So you work at the college?" she asked, already knowing the answer.

"Yes," I replied, "I just started about a month ago."

"My husband works there too," she said. "He runs the food service."

"Oh? I don't think I've met him yet." Technically the food service was outsourced to a giant corporation, but it meant he existed to serve the same students I ultimately served, so our fates were intertwined.

"I'll introduce you tonight at the bridge," she said, preparing to walk away. "Nice to meet you!"

"Ok, nice to meet you." I didn't know what bridge she meant.

Eliot said he wanted to go back on the bus with the team and would get himself home from the school. That seemed like a positive development in his social maturation process, even though I felt a little sad about it. After introducing myself to the coach, who thanked me for adding Eliot to the team, I headed home.

The light across the landscape had changed, now coming from overhead so there were no more long shadows among the farms. The car was warm and I felt sleepy, so I opted for the radio instead of another podcast. Options out in farm-land were limited: Christian music, country music, or classic rock. "Goodbye, stranger, it's been nice. Hope you find your paradise." I shut it off. Too on the nose.

When I got home, I allowed myself a proper nap of the sort I hadn't had since early in the summer—in my bed, in pajamas, under the covers, rather than merely tipped over haphazardly on the sofa. I dreamed of Eliot running and woke with a start when my phone dinged. My video text had finally gone through to Costa Rica and Moose had given it a thumbs-up. *You're welcome.*

When I went downstairs feeling sleep-drunk, Kelsey was on the sofa watching another episode of *Gilmore Girls*, which she had undoubtedly already seen dozens of times. I kissed her on the head.

"Hi hon. How you doing?"

"Bad. I miss my friends. They all went to a school dance last night."

"Aw, lovey, I'm sorry." I put my hands on her head and kissed her again. "Does your school have any dances coming up?"

"Yeah, next weekend. I'll probably go I guess." Her heart wasn't in it at the moment but I suspected by next week she'd be excited about it.

"If you want we can go dress shopping this week."

She perked up. "Really?"

"Sure! I'll ask Jamie about the best places to shop." It was nice to still be able to do things that made one of my kids happy.

In the kitchen I put some water on and ate a handful of peanuts (or two) while waiting for it to boil. I had meant to go to the grocery store on the way home from the meet, but in my torpor I'd forgotten. *Seriously, Jen, you need to figure out this shopping business. Your kids can't live on snacks alone.* I got some tea and sat down with Kelsey and my laptop to catch up on emails.

Before the tea had gotten cold, my taciturn boy came down the stairs.

"Can you give me a ride?"

I turned my stiff neck to look over my shoulder and blinked, as my brain toggled between a bad news email from the VP for Admissions (our final fall student count was down twelve percent from last fall) and the sound of my son's voice actually asking me for something.

He was wearing a slightly-too-large dress shirt and tie that I recognized as having once belonged to Moose, who apparently didn't need such items in Costa Rica. *Pura vida,* I scoffed inwardly. He smelled freshly showered and had product in his hair, making it look stiff and shiny.

"Right now?" I asked. He nodded. "Sure," I managed to answer, putting my laptop on the coffee table. "Where to?" It seemed much too early for a dance to start.

"We're meeting at the river bridge for pictures and then going to dinner." I remembered what Anna's mom had said earlier and shifted my brain back into mom mode.

"You and Anna?" His eyes grew wide and I grinned. "I met her mom at the meet this morning."

Resigned, his shoulders fell. "She's gonna drive us and her friends from there."

I could see how much it pained him to ask me for help because it meant I was going to be in public again, where I would be seen and interact with other people. My heart leaped at the chance to get a second rare glimpse into my kid's life. Then it sank when I realized I'd have to put my bra and jeans back on.

"OK, just give me a minute to make myself presentable," I said, standing up slowly and limping over to the stairs, as my body adjusted from being sedentary to being upright and moving again.

Upstairs I changed into real clothes, brushed my hair, splashed water on my face, and quickly brushed my teeth. I wiped the mascara circles from under my eyes and put lipstick on. I didn't look good, but definitely better. *Yesterday's eyeliner can be today's smoky eye if you believe in yourself.*

Downstairs Eliot and Kelsey were arguing because she wanted to go with us and he didn't want her along. "She can come," I said. He groaned and rolled his eyes but headed to the car, sitting shotgun and dutifully administering his seatbelt, avoiding all eye contact.

"So," I asked after we pulled out of the driveway, "What else can you tell me about Anna, besides that she's a runner?"

"Nothing," he sighed, "and please don't be embarrassing, OK? Just take your pictures and go." He turned to Kelsey in the backseat. "You too," he said.

"I'm never embarrassing," Kelsey said. "*You're* the weirdo in this family."

"Whatever."

When we got to the park I grabbed my mask and asked Eliot if he had one. "It's fine," he replied, getting out of the car. I could see that no one else there—neither the elegantly dressed kids nor their photo-shooting parents—was wearing one. *Did you really think the kids were going to wear masks to a dance?* Maybe the pandemic was over in St. Jutta. I gave silent thanks for vaccines, left my mask in the car, and hoped for the best. *When in Rome.*

I followed Eliot till he gravitated near a group of giggling girls by an old railroad trestle. Some were wearing full-length gowns, others in mini dresses threatening to expose their butt cheeks. One had hair long enough to sit on. Eliot didn't introduce me to anyone so I hovered nearby till I identified Anna's mom.

"Hi Amy," I said, approaching her as confidently as I could, despite feeling significantly older and frumpier than she was. Behind her was Anna in a short (but not butt-cheek short) sparkly dress that looked fit for a disco. Her braids had been replaced with long curls that she had probably been working on since leaving the meet. I was always in awe of people who could make their hair look like television hair.

"You must be Anna," I said.

"Yes, hi," she said with a little wave, grinning from ear to ear like a girl with a serious crush. Her eyes were warm and smart. I liked her immediately.

"I'm Jen," I said. "This is Kelsey."

"I love your dress!" Kelsey said effusively.

"Thanks," Anna answered. Below her knees was a pair of pink Chuck Taylors that echoed Eliot's red ones. *Oh my god, he found a girl who wants to wear matching shoes.* I thought I might die of cuteness overload. I wanted desperately to thank her for asking my boy to a dance and giving him his first taste of high school social life, but I thought that would definitely fall into the "embarrassing" category so I held my tongue.

The kids talked amongst themselves, the boys looking happy but awkward, the girls giddy with excitement like Bennett sisters before a ball at Netherfield. For a split second I could remember that feeling *exactly*, before it vanished just as quickly.

Amy said, "This is my husband, Jake." A short, barrel-chested man with a buzz cut offered his hand so I shook it.

While making a mental note to use hand sanitizer when I got back in the car (I didn't have time to get sick), I said, "Nice to meet you, Jake. I hear you work at the college too?"

"Yep, sixteen years this fall," he said. "Although technically, since two years ago, I don't work for the college anymore."

"Right," I said, unsure of how to read his tone. "How has it been since the change-over?"

"Terrible. The company slashed our budget so we're understaffed and undersupplied. And for the new employees, their kids don't even get free tuition anymore, which used to be the best thing about the job. I'm actually looking for other jobs now since Anna doesn't want to go to St. Margaret's anyway."

"Jake!" Amy said, alarmed. She looked at me apologetically.

"Oh, don't worry," I hurried to reassure her, "I'm not involved in those decisions and I won't tell." I did, however, make a mental note to bring up the outsourcing and understaffing at the next cabinet meeting. "I just started last month on the academic side of things."

"Yep."

"So where does Anna want to go to school?"

"Eastern Michigan University in Ypsilanti. She got a full ride for the four-year nursing bachelor's program." EMU, like the other regional state schools, was absolutely killing St. Margaret's with financial aid this year. We just couldn't compete for the state's dwindling supply of high school graduates. Or nursing faculty, for that matter.

"Wow, that's wonderful. As far as I know, Eliot hasn't even thought about college yet." I felt a tickle of anxiety growing in my chest so I changed the subject. "What about you, Amy?"

"I'm a nurse in an OB-GYN's office." She said "OB-gin" rather than spelling out the letters. I asked which one and made a mental note *not* to go there. I glanced over at Eliot to make sure I wasn't embarrassing him. He was engrossed in his companions and not looking at me.

"You know, Anna's been to lots of dances over the years," Amy said quietly, looking at her daughter, "but she's never asked a boy out before. Eliot must be very special."

"Aw thanks. I was thinking Anna must be special if she could actually see something in my boy." She looked horrified. *What kind of mother says a thing like that?* "Because he's usually so shy!"

"Oh, ok," she laughed. "Well Anna's not, obviously. She's a really safe driver, by the way."

"I'm sure she is. I told Eliot he has to pay for dinner since she's driving." We exchanged phone numbers just in case. It all felt very pleasant and I hoped Eliot would approve.

The kids started lining themselves up in a group and the parents started snapping pictures. When the group dispersed, Amy (bless her) insisted on getting some shots of the couple alone, which meant I could get some too. I was in awe as Eliot and Anna put their arms around each other so naturally. *Who is that well-adjusted boy?* Then Amy wanted a picture of the couple with their parents in it, so I handed my phone to Kelsey, and Eliot was forced to smile while I put my arm around him.

"OK, you can go now," he said under his breath when the picture had been taken. I thought I should quit while I was ahead, so I wished them all a good time and Kelsey and I went back to the car. I was on the verge of tears, feeling both happy and like there was a brick on my chest.

No one had warned me that having a teenage son would be so heartbreaking. I mourned the loss of my sweet little boy, the one who used to love me, who wanted to be around me, who was up for any activity I suggested, who needed my help and said cute things and generally brought light into my life. That baby was gone, lost to me and never coming back, and I grieved for him almost as if he were dead.

I also mourned over the big kid whom I so desperately wanted to know, but who didn't like me anymore. That feeling was almost like being dumped—like someone had broken up with me, but I still had to see him every day while he ignored me and hung out with his new friends. It was unrequited love. I still longed to hug him and tell him I loved him, while he could barely stand the sight of me. I was like some needy, creepy stalker he couldn't shake. Like a cast-off turd on the bottom of his shoe.

"I can't wait to go to high school," Kelsey said wistfully. "Can we get pizza tonight?" I put my arm around her and kissed her on top of the head, thanking the universe for giving me the most adorable distraction from my most de-pressing thought spirals.

We stopped to order a mediocre midwestern pie for takeout, and when we got home we did a bit of Facebook stalking on Anna and her family. Anna liked YA novels and Taylor Swift, so she met with Kelsey's approval. Amy mostly posted family photos, including a few of Anna and Eliot already (and the one all of us, in which I looked so hideous I wanted to cry). She and her husband had also recently celebrated their 20th anniversary, and to celebrate they'd held a 90s-themed prom at the St. Jutta high school, from which they had apparently both graduated. It made me nostalgic for my home state and the sense of belonging I had there.

As I tried to sleep that night, I couldn't stop wondering how I had gone from being the adorable girl in the homecoming photos to the embarrassing mom with the camera. And how had it happened so fast?

Chapter 10

A Very Good Girl

I have always been a good girl. I was an easy child for my parents, and teachers loved me. I did everything I was supposed to do and did it well, both at home and at school. At eighteen I was accepted to Wellesley, but my mom was so distraught at the idea of "losing me" to a place five hours away that I chose Madison College instead—a second-tier school but only a half hour's drive.

I flourished there—friends, grades, orchestra, all good. I fell in love with Italian so I double-majored in modern languages and history and did a spring semester abroad in Genoa. In the fall of my senior year, my professor convinced me to go on to graduate school. In the early 90s it wasn't such a stupid idea; the nation's broader job market was terrible and higher education seemed stable in comparison, flush with cash and students. Plus my boyfriend of two years had dumped me in Rome over spring break, so any marriage plans I might have nurtured about being a young bride were dead. I needed a Plan B.

I went to a PhD program at Princeton, met Moose, and was off on the academic fast track—dissertation completed and tenure-track job secured at 27, tenured at 33 (perhaps less impressive than Jesus, but it felt important at the time), full professor at 39, and finally, holder of the Miles J. Benedict, Jr. Chair of Modern Languages. At 42 I was the youngest Madison professor, as well as the first woman, ever to hold an endowed chair in any field. I was not only a good girl, I was apparently a trailblazer.

But after that, things stalled out, professionally. There was nowhere for me to go, no more worlds to conquer. I had chaired all the important committees and the faculty senate. I had built good relationships with my bosses and had sat on countless (mostly pointless) task forces with presidents and vice presidents. For a while I convinced myself that stagnation wasn't such a bad thing, that it was a good time to rest on my laurels a little bit. I had done what I came here to do and could now find some balance—focus on my kids while they were still young, spend more time with my family, and maybe read for fun or even exercise now and then.

But I was bored.

Moose, tired of my complaining (and bored himself, I realized in hindsight), convinced me I should try to get a job in administration. I spent a three-year term as part-time dean at Madison. Then I applied for a handful of dean, director, and provost positions all across the country in the fall of 2019, got a couple of first interviews, and made it to a campus interview in February 2020 at St. Margaret's. You know the rest.

So now, at almost 52, here I was: the Plan B Provost and Vice President for Academic Affairs at the College of St. Margaret.

People were shocked when I left Madison, a nationally-known, well-respected liberal arts college with a 750 million-dollar endowment, a cool location, and even a few famous alumni. It was a safety school for wealthy East Coast kids who didn't get into the Ivy Leagues or who wanted to live near New York City—a pretty lucrative niche to fill, even in hard economic times. Madison College wasn't immune to the 21st-century struggles of higher education, but it was pretty well insulated from the very worst financial symptoms.

St. Margaret's, on the other hand, was a regional college that no one in New Jersey had heard of, co-ed but still disproportionately female, with an endowment of only about $90,000,000. More than three-quarters of its students were from Michigan, a state rapidly losing population, and the rest mostly from Ohio, with a handful of football players from Texas and Florida. (Division III schools technically can't offer athletics scholarships, but they offer a lot of "merit-based" aid to the students they really want, including athletes.) About a third of St. Margaret's students were eligible for Pell grants, and exactly none of them paid anything close to full tuition, which was already $25,000 lower than Madison's outrageous sticker price. A few students had mothers or grandmothers who were alumni, but lots of students had parents who hadn't been to college at all.

Young people picked St. Margaret's for pretty much three reasons: to get a degree in business, nursing, or a pre-health discipline; to play four more years of sports; and/or because St. Margaret's offered a private education that, with "discounts," ended up costing the same as a public one. Needless to say, the college couldn't afford to offer any Italian, and even as a senior administrator my new salary here was only marginally better than my old one. (I literally shuddered when I found out how little the two tenured Spanish professors earned, after the Faculty Women's Caucus had complained about salary inequities.) It was almost like living in another country. I could see firsthand how the rich got richer while everyone else fought for leftovers.

But to get back to me—I was, for the first time in my life, finding it really hard to know how to be a good girl.

Sitting in the Provost's seat, I wasn't sure whom to please. Norm Festerling, the college president, was my boss. Ultimately he could fire me, so at an obvious level I needed to make sure he was happy with my performance. In the past, I had been highly adept at making my superiors love me because I had always been competent and reliable and didn't make waves, even when I rarely expressed occasional dissent. Though I didn't yet feel competent in my provost role, I had confidence that I would become competent soon enough. But many of my values were much more aligned with the faculty than with the administration. If I wanted to please my boss, I would have to quell some of my habitual, faculty-centric reactions in favor of the bigger picture.

And yet, the faculty also needed pleasing—as my predecessor discovered the hard way. Unhappy faculty were bad for everyone, especially students, but also provosts. Faculty couldn't fire anyone, but they could talk to HR or the president any time they wanted, and if they were really determined to get rid of me, they could take a no-confidence vote in a faculty meeting. Meanwhile, my authority over them was very limited. Technically speaking, tenured faculty can be fired, but only after months' or years' worth of procedures (unless they did something truly egregious and illegal, like grope a student or shout racist epithets at a colleague). Truth be told, I tended to side with the faculty on most things, having spent more than two decades as one of them. But as Provost, I wasn't supposed to *tell* them when I sided with them.

So I was now walking a knife's edge between satisfying my boss or satisfying the faculty, without dissatisfying the other too terribly.

Today was one of those knife-edge days. The leadership had a budget meeting. I had to figure out how to tell my boss what he wanted to hear about cutting costs in the academic sector, when what I really wanted to tell him was how badly we needed a significant *increase* in our budget if we were to keep offering students anything close to (what I considered to be) a high-quality undergraduate degree. After two years of hybrid and masked teaching, and now struggling with students who had lost almost two years of education, social development, and mental health, the faculty—like the high school teachers and guidance counselors they had basically become—were hanging at the ends of their utterly frayed ropes. They needed rest. They needed to feel appreciated.

They needed raises.

So when the president announced that he and the board had decided that sabbaticals had to go, in the same meeting where he had just announced million-dollar renovations to the football stadium, my head almost exploded. My face grew hot and my hands started to jitter as he offered his rationale about how sabbaticals were a thing of the past, when colleges were on top of the world and could afford to pay professors enough to maintain an upper middle-class lifestyle.

And when most professors were white men with wives at home, I resisted interjecting.

"Today's colleges need to be leaner and more agile," he concluded, as the COO and CFO nodded in approval. I could practically see them working his marionette strings.

"That's a terrible idea," I said before thinking. *Shit.* My filter lately was not functioning up to its usual level.

"I'm sorry?"

"Sorry," I smiled, trying to regroup and adopt a rational tone, "but have you thought about how this will affect our ability to attract and retain the best faculty? The promise of a sabbatical tends to be a big draw at hiring time." My filter now back on, I did not add: *Rural Michigan is a hard sell, so we need all the help we can get.*

"Yes, we absolutely want to maintain a top-notch faculty," he said, "and as you know, it's a buyer's market in most fields nowadays."

My hackles went up. I knew by "most fields" he meant my beloved humanities and social sciences, now seen as superfluous luxury items by many Americans. But I decided to be strategic and focus on the things I knew he cared about.

"It's not a 'buyer's market' in business or nursing," I said. "We are already struggling to find and keep enough faculty in those departments, even part-time. And I have to pay full-time adjuncts almost as much as tenured faculty."

"Yes," he said, "we absolutely need to be able to pay nurses and business experts what they're worth if we want to remain fully staffed. I'm grateful that so many of our board members have stepped up to teach business classes." *Purely out of the goodness of their hearts, I'm sure.*

"That money has to come from somewhere," the COO added unhelpfully. My cheeks burned and my armpits felt like tiny jacuzzies.

"So," I said, pausing for a breath and trying to tread carefully, "is our strategy to take money from the humanities and social sciences, which provide courses that every St. Margaret's student has to take to graduate, in order to lure nurses and business professors away from their 'real' jobs?" The devil on my shoulder said, *If they were any good at nursing or business, they wouldn't be looking to teach at a third-tier college anyway.*

"Their time is extremely valuable," Norm said, "and we have to make it worth their while."

"So, are we saying it's OK to..." (I was going to say "exploit" but thought better of it) "underpay highly-qualified faculty in fields where the supply of PhDs outstrips the number of jobs, in order to use those savings to overpay teachers in other fields, who are both less qualified and less committed to educating young people?"

No one answered. People still didn't know me that well and weren't sure how to read my tone. I kept going.

"Maybe not everyone here knows this, but we already pay part-time nurses and business instructors, most of whom have, at most, a master's degree or 'relevant experience,' $6,000 per course. That's compared to the $3,000 that adjuncts with PhDs get for teaching in the liberal arts departments. They are definitely not doing twice as much work as other instructors do, and frankly paying them more does not guarantee that they are any good at teaching. And meanwhile," *oh my god, someone please interrupt me*, "every

St. Margaret's student—including nursing and business majors—has to take multiple humanities, arts, and social science courses to fulfill the general education requirements that we promise will make them 'well-rounded.' So this means those divisions are *already* subsidizing the business and nursing majors."

"Yes, in fact I've already been in conversations with the board about spinning off business and nursing into their own schools," the president said.

Are you even listening to me? I wanted to shout. Instead I said, "I'm afraid we're starving the liberal arts out of this liberal arts college."

That was too much for the COO. He was the retired CEO of some small-time manufacturing company, still relatively new to academia and unaccustomed to seeing subordinates talk to their bosses this way.

"Jennifer," he held out a hand to stop me, "liberal arts is a non-starter these days. We are now a 'regional college' according to U.S. News." He made finger quotes. All eyes were on him. "If we're gonna stay afloat we have to give customers what they want. Customers don't care about 'liberal arts' or who teaches their philosophy classes."

The president, a philosophy PhD, flinched but didn't interrupt.

"They only care if they can get a job when they graduate," the COO went on. "So yes, we're gonna do whatever we have to do to save money on the products customers don't value, and we're gonna invest in the products they do value. That's how markets work."

I sat in stunned silence, out of moves. *He just said the quiet part out loud.*

"It's just reality," he added, shaking his head and throwing up his hands, done trying to reason with me.

"Yes," Norm finally broke in, "it's very important that we stay attuned to our students' needs in the current economic climate." I could see him trying to rephrase the COO's speech into something a bit more palatable. "Of course, they also need soft skills like writing and critical thinking and global awareness, in addition to more specific job skills, and St. Margaret's will continue to provide all of that for them, to the extent that we can afford to do so."

I had so much more I wanted to say, but I felt defeated. *You know this is how it is, Jen. Only the very richest schools can afford to keep the liberal arts fully funded and fully staffed with well-qualified faculty. You just forgot how lucky you were to be at Madison. Don't make enemies just yet.*

As the meeting moved on, I focused on my breathing and made a mental note to look for ways to optimize the academic budget as soon as possible. I also planned to buy some of those women's undershirts with built-in armpit bras.

Chapter 11

Fall Semester Blues

The rest of the fall semester was a total blur. My allergies were horrible for months. Something about Michigan's autumn didn't agree with me. So now in addition to leaking from all my other orifices, I also leaked constantly from my nose. I started hiding tissues in my sleeves like my grandma. I could hardly wait for the first hard frost.

At work I did my best not to be the worst. I got to my office by 8:00 a.m. every day. I rushed around from meeting to meeting—with the cabinet, with the president, with the registrar, with the librarians, with various faculty governance committees—all the things that fell into my rather broad column. I attended a Sukkoth event with the college's two Jewish students and three Jewish professors. I made a presentation to the board of trustees and schmoozed at the college's homecoming reunion. I never felt fully prepared for almost anything I had to do, but somehow I kept going—*fake it till you make it*—and everyone was polite enough not to remark upon my many areas of ignorance.

In between meetings outside my office, I welcomed a steady stream of people into my office for confidential meetings—anxious or disgruntled faculty, staff, and students who usually wanted to complain about their mean department chairs, their mean colleagues, or their mean professors. Such complaints were familiar to me, being the same kinds of things people complained about at Madison over the years. But now that I was in the provost's chair they hit me a bit differently. Sometimes, especially when dealing with tenured faculty, I wished they would just grow up and talk to their tormentors directly like grown-ass adults. Other times, when there was a genuine power differential at play, I felt as if I should be able to fix things.

And yet when it came to actually providing solutions, I couldn't quite figure out how to address problems in a way that wouldn't simply make them worse. I didn't want to step on anyone's toes or come across as dictatorial, or inadvertently bring down retribution on bullies' underlings. At some point, certain issues might require provost action, but until I was sure, I tried to slow-walk my involvement by suggesting actions the plaintiffs could try themselves.

An exception was the question of faculty salaries, which was an area where I actually had some authority. As they had promised me back in August, the Women's Caucus (which I had since learned was not an actual college organization but simply four angry women) put salary inequity on the October faculty meeting agenda. They had put a one-page resolution into the meeting packet, in which several WHEREAS statements led to a THEREFORE. That much was unremarkable.

What was remarkable was that the THEREFORE proposal was to make all faculty salaries public, like they are at public universities, and that they had all signed off with their names and shamefully small salaries.

Vivian, $64,450, spoke for the group, while the others sat in the front row for moral support. She stood, tall and straight, in the front of the lecture hall, a silk scarf draped around her enviably swan-like neck. "I know you can all read so I won't bother reading the resolution. I will be glad to answer any questions."

For a moment it seemed no one had anything to say. Then a dozen hands went up. The faculty chair called on a middle-aged biologist—another WMB—first.

"I am utterly against this proposal," he said, already red in the face. "It's it's it's... my salary is private and it's nobody's fucking business what I make." As he spoke, I recalled that his base salary was a good $20,000 more than Vivian's, not including any research grants he got. "I have a PhD, I've been here twenty-three years, and I work hard to earn my salary."

"I also work hard to earn my salary," Vivian said calmly. "And while I don't have a PhD, I do have a terminal degree in my field and I've been here thirty years." *How is she not sweating right now?* The faculty chair called on an associate professor of history.

"I appreciate that it is unfair that some of us earn much less than others, even when we've worked the same amount of time and have the same degree," she said, "but making our salaries public is not the best way to create equality. This is a matter for the administration, and for private conversations between faculty and the Provost." She looked at me. *Oh right, that's me.* I arranged my face into what I hoped was a serious-but-friendly smile. "Making our salaries public will only cause comparison and division among us."

"We submit that there is already comparison and division among us," Vivian responded. "Those of us who are underpaid are well aware that we are underpaid because there is aggregated data available in the *Chronicle of Higher Education*. Secrecy about our salaries only benefits the administration and those with above-average salaries."

"Frankly, my salary is so low that I would be embarrassed for everyone to know about it," said a young art professor with a nervous laugh. "Can't I just live in my happy bubble and be grateful I have a job at all?"

"You probably deserve better," Vivan told her.

The conversation went on for about a half hour, before an elderly math professor called for a vote. The resolution failed, by about three to one. I didn't think the Women's Caucus had actually expected it to pass, but I had to admire the fact that they'd gotten people talking about it. And it gave me an excuse to take it to the President—who was sitting in the far back corner of the room, looking relieved.

Sometimes in the middle of the workday I would get so exhausted I almost couldn't see straight, but I was afraid to sneak a power nap in my office because of the time Fran caught me dozing with my head on the desk. So one day I tried to sneak a nap in this weird storage area between the faculty lounge and the all-gender restroom. There was an old forest green pleather bench hidden behind some stacked filing cabinets, and if I curled up fetal-style I could be hidden from any casual passers-through. I had just ducked out of consciousness when I was brought back by two people, mid-conversation, as they entered the lounge.

A woman's voice that I didn't initially recognize said, "Well at least they fired the last guy. He really was the worst."

"Oh no," said a man's gravelly voice, this one unmistakably belonging to the British religious studies professor nearing retirement, who had questioned me disapprovingly during my interview two years ago, "my philosophy is, things always get worse."

She laughed. "How could she possibly be worse than a serial harasser?" I now recognized the speaker as the anthropologist, slowly awaking to the fact that the "she" in that sentence was me.

"It remains to be seen," he said quietly, "but I've been here long enough to know that every new administrator is more craven and incompetent than the last. It's just the way the modern university is going now. Good people get chewed up and spit out, and those who remain are those who do exactly what their corporate overlords tell them to do." I could practically hear him shaking his head.

"Well I hope you're wrong," she said.

"Yes, I suppose I hope so too," he replied.

Me too, dude, me too.

That particular night, when I dragged myself past St. Margaret on my way home, she was just a statue staring blankly into the distance, offering no words of wisdom for a new, inexperienced boss just doing her best. *Fine. Thanks for nothing.*

Much of the time I was grumpy due to being desperately in need of sleep, which lately I couldn't seem to get. Even when I managed to fall asleep, I'd be wide awake and sweaty an hour later. Gone were the days when I could function on five or six hours. I briefly thought about my banished CPAP, but then banished that thought, not wanting to give Moose the satisfaction, even in absentia. I wondered if he wore it with Amber, or if she was still honeymoonish enough to put up with his snoring.

After another dinner of spaghetti with store-bought sauce and baby carrots ("You should really buy real carrots that don't come in a plastic bag," Eliot said), I went into my bathroom to brush my teeth. When I turned on the light I was assaulted by the mess. It wasn't new; it had been growing for days or weeks, but there never seemed to be a good time to clean. Now I felt disgust at the soap scum on the shower door and the cat-hair-covered toilet and the grimy sink and the explosion of personal care products covering the counter. And I didn't even have a partner to share the blame.

For a moment I considered turning off the light and going straight to bed, but the horror was now burned into my brain and I wouldn't rest till I dealt with it. I got out the toxic chemicals to kill the grout mold, sprayed it on, and then breathed through my mouth while putting items away in drawers and the medicine cabinet. Meanwhile my colleague's words, "Things always get worse," ran on a loop in my head.

While I was hunched over, scrubbing the toilet, Eliot appeared in the doorway looking as if he had something on his mind.

"Hi, hon," I said, glad of the interruption. "What's up?"

"Anna is coming over to watch *The Book of Boba Fett* on Saturday," he said. I gawked at him. Then with a perfectly straight face he added, "You have to be somewhere else."

I hadn't entirely finished processing part one of his announcement before he added part two, and my brain was short-circuiting.

My kid? Invited a girl to our house? And he wants to be alone with her? *He is seventeen, Jen*, said my wiser self. *You should have anticipated this.*

"Hello?" Eliot said, annoyed. I closed my gaping mouth and composed myself.

"You are welcome to have a friend over on Saturday," I said as lightly as I could. "I won't be leaving the house but I promise to leave you alone." He threw his head back and rolled his eyes. "But I need you to please help me clean before she comes. We don't want her to see the slovenly pit we currently call home."

We were going to have to do a thorough cleaning before my parents came for Thanksgiving anyway, because I couldn't let my mother see how much my housekeeping skills had devolved. There were still a few boxes we hadn't unpacked sitting in the corner of the dining room. I honestly had no idea what was in there.

"Ugh, fine," he replied.

To his credit, Eliot did spend most of that Saturday helping me clean the house. He even set his alarm for 10:00 a.m. to give himself plenty of time. At around 3:30 he got in the shower where he spent the better part of the next hour. I drove Kelsey to her friend's for a sleepover. By 5:00, when he came down and began pacing near the front window, the public areas—living room, dining room, kitchen, and powder room—were looking nice, almost as if we were the kind of family that kept the house clean. If she stuck around she would eventually find out the truth, but there was no need to introduce it too soon.

"She's here," he said quietly as I was emptying the dishwasher.

"Ok," I said. "Let her in."

He looked at me seriously and made a gesture with his hands pushing the air downward, as if to say, "Be cool." I nodded in agreement. *Seriously, Jen, be cool.*

I waited in the kitchen while he greeted her at the door. I heard her stop to pat Fiona, who was always curious about newcomers. A few moments later they entered the kitchen and I was reminded of a phrase I'd once read, about walking as close to someone as you could get "without it being a three-legged race." She stayed right behind him, as if in need of protection.

I welcomed her warmly, asked her about school, and offered her a drink. She chit-chatted with me and showed me a picture of her cat. She looked adorable and smelled good, having obviously put a lot of effort into her appearance even for a night of TV watching, with shimmery eyeshadow and her long hair curled just so.

Wow, she must really like him, I thought.

Why does that surprise you? I thought back.

I dunno, maybe because he's a total jerk to me most of the time?

Speaking of being a jerk, Eliot started signaling to me with his eyeballs that it was time for me to go. We had agreed that I could stay long enough to say hello but then I had to disappear into the office-guestroom or upstairs. I excused myself and headed to the office with the promise (also pre-approved) to order them a pizza in a couple of hours. While I worked, I could hear them occasionally laughing, which delighted me and also made me feel strangely homesick.

When I went out to tell them the pizza was coming, they were sitting close to each other on the sofa under the faux fur blanket, Fiona fast asleep on Anna's lap. A train on the TV rode through a desert, being attacked by people on speeders. Eliot acknowledged me briefly over his shoulder. I quickly entered the kitchen, fixed myself a peanut butter sandwich and a cup of tea (thinking I should refrain from drinking alcohol while someone else's child was under my care), and carried them upstairs along with my laptop just as Eliot was answering the door for the pizza delivery. I had left a five dollar bill by the door and instructed him to hand it to the driver, since who knew what tips they actually got from those delivery apps we all used now.

I spent the next few hours intermittently working, checking social media, and straining to listen for signs of life downstairs. Around eleven I was feeling sleepy and wanted to go to bed but Anna was still there. It hadn't occurred to me to talk about a curfew—we'd never been in this situation before. When I walked across the hall to the bathroom and looked down the stairs, I noticed it was dark and quiet, though I could still see some flickering light on the walls from the TV.

Yikes, I thought. *What do I do now?*

A terrifying thought occurred to me.

<Hi, Moose. Did you ever have the condom talk with Eliot?> It was an hour earlier in Costa Rica so I figured he would still be awake.

<No> he wrote back a minute later. Then <???>.

<He has a girl over. [mind-blown emoji]>

<Good for him>

Way to act like a man, man. I typed an angry emoji and then deleted it.

<It's almost midnight and the lights are off! [Anxious emoji]>

<They'll be fine stop worrying>

And that was it. As far as I could tell I had two choices: interrupt their evening or trust them. I decided to trust them, since they were both about to fly their respective nests anyway.

While lying in bed fretting, I somehow drifted off to sleep until I woke to the sound of the front door closing. My phone said it was 2:15 a.m. As I heard Eliot quietly creeping up the stairs I made a mental note to have the condom talk with him tomorrow.

Yeah, he's gonna love that.

I wondered why I hadn't done it sooner, except that I always thought I'd have more time. We had taught him about "making babies" when he was very little, and we had never been secretive about sex. Between that and whatever they taught him in health class, I was confident he knew the mechanics. But I had definitely planned to talk to him about contraception and consent before he left for college, or whenever he got his first serious girlfriend. Anna had seemingly come out of nowhere. What if it was already too late? *Please, universe, don't let it be too late.*

Meanwhile, there was occasional drama in my easy child's life. On the Friday before Halloween, Kelsey got contact-traced at school and was told she had to stay home for a week. She was devastated, not because she might be sick, but because I said she couldn't go to a Halloween sleepover party with her new friends on Saturday. (The town had set hours on Saturday evening when kids could go trick-or-treating, even though Halloween fell on Sunday.) She was furious with me and slammed herself into her bedroom—heretofore a rare occurrence—apparently to call her friend, whose mother called me a few minutes later.

When the phone rang, I was hugging an ice pack in front of the freezer to try to cool down after my daughter's tantrum, and didn't answer because I didn't recognize the number. A moment later my phone dinged. A voice straight out of *Fargo* had left a message.

"Hi, this is Avery's mom. I just wanted to let you know that I know Kelsey got contact-traced at school..." (she pronounced it *can-tact*) "but we're not worried about it and she's welcome to come to Avery's sleepover tomorrow if she wants to. Um, so, feel free to call me back if you want. Ok thanks, bye." I listened to the message again to catch her name, but she hadn't actually told me.

Why does no one here care about the pandemic? Am I the asshole?

"Kels," I knocked lightly on her door. "Kels, I need to talk to you."

A sullen teen with puffy eyes opened the door and stared at me. For a moment, before her features arranged themselves back into the familiar pattern in my brain, she looked like someone I didn't know.

"I heard from Avery's mom."

"So?"

"She doesn't care that you got contact-traced."

"I know, that's because Trinity got contact-traced too."

"Trinity?" I was still occasionally surprised by Gen Z names. I wondered if it was a Christian thing or a *Matrix* reference.

"Yeah, Trinity's going to Avery's too."

"So you're telling me that Avery's mom is letting her have a slumber party even though multiple guests might have Covid?" I was feeling judgmental and failing to hide it. I was also pissed off at Avery's mom for making me look like a paranoid meanie.

"Mo-oom," she stomped her foot, "it's called a sleepover, and no one has Covid!"

"You don't know that, sweetie."

"Yes I do!"

"No, you don't."

"And anyway, I'm young and I got vaccinated so I'll be fine!"

"A vaccine isn't magic, Kels!" I surprised myself by shouting, but I felt irritated with her self-centeredness, age-appropriate though it was. "And even if *you* don't get very sick, you might give it to me, and *I* might get really sick and I just don't have time for that right now. People my age who get Covid randomly drop dead of strokes and heart-attacks sometimes. Or get stuck in the hospital for weeks."

Her facial expression changed from tragedy to alarm. "They do?"

"Not always, but sometimes, yes. There's just no way to know how badly it's going to hit someone because it's different for everybody."

"Well..." she looked uncertain.

"I'm sorry, hon, but I can't let you go." She sighed but didn't protest anymore. "I promise you can have your friends over once everyone is in the clear."

The next day Kelsey told me that Avery had come down with a fever and a sore throat and her party was canceled. I was sorry for Avery but relieved to be back in my kid's good graces. The day after that, we got an early-morning automated phone message saying that there was a large outbreak in the middle school and all classes would be held virtually for the next two weeks. When I told Kelsey, she did a little happy dance because she hated being left out.

I looked out the window behind her and there was the most delicate snow falling, sometimes straight down, sometimes blowing gently sideways, first left, then right, like a cartoon or a movie set. Most of the trees had already dropped their leaves, but a clump of bright yellow ones clung to the gingko in Jamie's yard, and the puffy bushes in front of our porch (whose name I didn't know—Moose had been the gardener in the family) were still brilliant red.

I sat down on her bed for a minute to watch outside. Fiona came over and checked me out, finally making herself comfortable on my lap and starting to buzz. Snow falling always gave me the nostalgic urge to turn on the soundtrack from *A Charlie Brown Christmas*. I let myself play it on repeat every December, but never before.

In early November, the chaplain held a small Diwali event in support of our single Indian student. A few days after that, I learned about another holiday, this one particular to Michigan.

I was working in my office with the door open when I suddenly heard Fran gasp in the bay. My mom instincts propelled me toward the sound, but I stopped short when I saw a large man in overalls, Carhartt beanie, and plaid jacket, who appeared to be covered in blood. For a brief moment I thought we were under attack.

"Dear!" Fran whisper-yelled, "what are you doing here?"

"I locked myself out," he said.

"For heaven's sake, look at you!" she said, now glancing nervously at her boss, who was standing agape in the doorway. I was relieved we weren't being attacked but still confused about what was happening.

"Sorry, peach. If you give me the keys I'll get going." He smiled at me and said hi as Fran dug frantically through her massive purse.

Peach?

"Sorry," Fran said to me, "this is my husband, Jason."

"Hi," I said, shaking myself out of it. I wasn't sure if I should smile or look concerned, so I attempted a combination of both. "Is... everything ok?"

"Yeah, it's just opening day," she explained.

"Opening day?"

"Deer hunting," he answered cheerfully, "with regular firearms. Bow-hunting was last month."

I mouthed a silent "oh." Fran was ready for him to disappear.

"Goodbye," she said pointedly, handing him her keys. "Be sure to wash them off and hang them up by the door when you're done." She hurried him out the door. Jason and I waved our goodbyes and nice-to-meet-yous and he was gone. She checked her person to see if he had contaminated her with his bloody paws, and then took out a Lysol wipe to clean the doorknob.

"Sorry," she explained when she was done. Pumping some hand gel into her palm and vigorously rubbing her hands together, she added, "He looks forward to opening day all year."

I said nothing, still processing, so she went on.

"It's almost like Christmas for him and his brothers. He has a timer on his phone that counts down the days and hours all year long. They all went to his dad's house last night and slept over in their clothes so they could be in the woods at 3:00 this morning." She said this with an affectionate laugh, as if she knew it was weird but it also made her proud.

"Do you..." I desperately wanted to take advantage of this rare moment of self-disclosure between us but I had absolutely nothing to add to the conversation. I figured I'd try anyway. "Do you eat a lot of venison?" *Shit, do people even really call it venison?*

"Of course! We usually get a freezer full and he cooks it all year."

"Wow," I said.

"I can bring you some," she offered.

"Oh! Thanks!" I replied, too enthusiastically, hoping she would forget. Then again, maybe it would buy me some cred with my kid. He always said the only people who should eat meat are the ones who actually kill and process it themselves.

Not long after opening day, Kelsey's science teacher told her there was to be a partial lunar eclipse in the wee hours of the morning. She really wanted to see it, but her "fun" parent who would normally have enabled such things was in Costa Rica. I didn't want to let her down, so I had her sleep in my bed that night and we set an alarm for 4:00 a.m. I figured she would want to sleep through it when the time came, but it turned out I was projecting.

"Mom!" she was whisper-shouting and shaking me by the shoulder.

"What?" My heart pounded and for a moment I didn't recognize my bedroom.

"The eclipse! Come on!"

I groaned but wiped the crust off my face (my new bite guard exacerbated the problem) and got out of bed. We put on our slippers and coats and went out the front door. We walked into the street and looked southwest, and there it was, a lovely blob of a moon in an overcast sky, almost completely shaded except for a sliver of yellow-white on one side.

"Whoa!" she said.

"Yeah." The cold air was bracing but felt good in my lungs. Clean. I shivered and breathed deeply through my nostrils.

"That's Orion right?" She pointed at the constellation standing guard just to the moon's left.

"Yep, a giant hunter who was either the son of Poseidon and a human woman or, depending on whom you ask, made from a wineskin filled with the urine of the gods and buried underground for nine months."
"Eeuwww, Mom!"

"That's how the myth goes," I said matter-of-factly. "The Romans thought his name sounded like their word for urine." *He was also reputedly a rapist but that was par for the course back in the day.* "There's a fountain dedicated to him in Sicily."

"A peeing fountain?"

"No, just a regular fountain. There is a peeing fountain in Brussels called *Manneken Pis*. Little boy pissing."

"Gross."

The street was quiet and still. A couple of houses had porch lights on. Jamie's pride flags waved almost imperceptibly. Puffs of breath floated out of us. Kelsey leaned close to me and I put my arms around her.

I felt totally peaceful for a few moments before remembering the countless horrors going on in the world, even as we admired the moon. I never used to dwell on depressing stuff, but for some reason lately I couldn't seem to shake the thought that I'd brought my children into a shit-show of a world, and that someday I would leave them there to figure it out without my help. A now-familiar sinking feeling punched me in the chest.

Jesus, Jen, you really know how to ruin a beautiful moment.

Chapter 12

Giving Thanks or Whatever

My parents had been planning to spend the week of Thanksgiving with us, but their trip was delayed when my dad fainted and ended up spending Saturday night in the hospital. The root problem turned out to be a fairly advanced urinary tract infection that had given him a fever. He had of course failed to mention any symptoms to my mom or his doctor until it was too late. They treated it with IV antibiotics, and because he was also on blood thinners and had hit his head when falling, they wanted to keep an eye on him. So they missed their Sunday flight.

They still wanted to come, but at that late date, the best available replacement flights were on Thanksgiving morning. I felt guilty for being relieved about having four fewer nights to host them and resolved to make sure their shortened stay was extra special.

That Monday, my phone rang at five in the morning. I awoke in a panic, but it was only an automated message from the schools, announcing a two-hour delay due to "ice and fog." I tried to go back to sleep but the adrenaline had already taken hold in my system, so I figured I'd get some work done.

I got up and looked out the window. It was still dark. The fog put Chapel Street in soft focus. I went to Kelsey's room and turned off her phone alarm, and texted Eliot about the delay. (It had been a long time since I dared touch his phone.)

I took a quick shower, put on pants and a blouse, and combed my wet hair. My head was cold but it felt good so I skipped the blow-dryer. I went quietly downstairs to the kitchen, washed out the coffeemaker, and started a fresh pot. While it brewed, I fed Fiona, loaded the dishwasher, cleaned off the counters, and emptied the trash can, which was overflowing thanks to Eliot's most recent Oreo package.

I sighed. Periodically, I warned my son that no one else in his life would ever love him enough to clean up his messes day after day, but my warnings hadn't yet inspired him to become a better roommate. Thus, my choices were either to let things go to shit, or to clean up after him and maintain some semblance of my sanity. So clean up after him I often did.

I picked the biggest mug in the cupboard, the one that said "My 50th birthday: the one where I was quarantined," which my sister-in-law had given me in 2020, back when we were still sisters-in-law, and back when we thought the pandemic was going to be just a few-week thing. I got my laptop from the kitchen table and went to the sofa, where I sat in the dark under a blanket. Fiona sat near me on the armchair giving herself a post-breakfast bath.

The next hour or so I dedicated to answering emails from faculty (someone kept leaving classroom desks in a circle instead of rows in room 109 – *the horror!*), fellow administrators (a few student-athletes were still on academic probation and needed prompt re-review following mid-term grading), and the president (mostly forwarded emails from trustees, faculty, and students about academic matters that were my purview). I could have easily made email my full-time job. I wished I could let Fran handle some of it, but I wasn't confident in her de-escalation skills.

Later, as the kids were getting breakfast and I was putting on makeup, another automated call came announcing school was canceled altogether. When I told them, Kelsey did a happy dance before plopping herself in front of the TV. Eliot went back upstairs without comment.

"Are you gonna be ok, hon?" I said to Kelsey. "I still have to go to work."

"I'll be fine," she said as Netflix bleeped-blooped. I sighed. I felt guilty leaving her at home with no one but the TV, a cat, and a surly teenage boy for company, but it couldn't be helped. I kissed the top of her head. "Take good care of her, Fiona."

I was first to arrive in the office that day, pleased with myself for making it in on the slick sidewalks without falling. (I kept thinking about that "Black Ice" sketch on *Key & Peele*.) Fran came in a few minutes late, looking upset and apologizing profusely.

"Is everything ok?"

"The roads are just terrible," she answered, putting down her bags and brushing the snow out of her hair. "I almost ran into a ditch." I had been informed that the college almost never closed for weather since pretty much all the students lived on campus. Never mind that more than half of our employees commuted from well out of town.

"I was wondering about that," I said, helping her with her coat. "Why don't we just go virtual when the weather is this dangerous?"

"The COO says people have to come in person or they won't do their work." We had a Cabinet meeting later that day so I made a mental note to ask about reevaluating our weather policy.

As it happened, when I got to the conference room there were only three of us there—me, the President, and the diversity and inclusion director. Everyone else was calling in from home due to the weather. Their disembodied voices floated in through the black plastic octopus in the middle of the table. A surge of righteous anger pumped through my veins.

"I'm glad you can all stay home and be safe," I said before the meeting had officially started, channeling my inner diplomat and looking at Norm. "It would be great if faculty and staff could also stay home on days like today. Fran had a horrible time getting here this morning." Norm shifted in his chair. "I'm not sure it makes sense to put employees' lives in danger when we've proven to ourselves over the past couple of years that most things can be done remotely if needed."

It was the COO who answered. "The hourly staff need to come in if they want to get paid," he said. "There's just no way to make sure they're doing their jobs if they're not here."

I was glad he wasn't, in fact, "here" so he couldn't see my reaction to the irony of his statement. His toxic managerial philosophy, imported from the for-profit world, suddenly gave me a vision of those parasitoid wasps that lay their eggs inside other insects, their spawn slowly killing their hosts from the inside out as they grow.

"Faculty are not hourly staff," I said calmly, conscious of the heat rising in my cheeks, "but I suspect even most hourly staff can be trusted to do their work at home, as much as anyone else can." Then, against my better judgment, I added, "And anyway, I'm not sure how you can make sure folks are working if you're not even here to supervise them." *What are you doing, Jen?*

"Yes," Norm interjected quickly, "we want to make sure that everyone in our community is safe. Jennifer, the academic sector is your sector, so by all means, feel free to set appropriate policies for faculty and other academic staff." *Artfully played, Norm.*

"Great. I'll work with the personnel committee to figure out what works."

A phone dinged and I realized it was mine, with Kelsey's tone. "Sorry, this is my daughter," I said. Looking down, I saw a selfie of Kelsey and Jamie smiling ear to ear, red-cheeked and in the snow. "SLEDDING," read the text.

The warm feeling in my face suddenly felt pleasant rather than menacing. I wondered if there was a special term for a trans Manic Pixie Dream Girl who sponsored a single mom and her kids. That thought made me feel guilty, so I made a mental note to ask Jamie over soon. I quickly texted her as the CFO droned on about three-year projections.

<<THANK YOU! [snowflake][sled][heart][grateful hands] I owe you!>>

On Thanksgiving morning, Kelsey and I made the trek to Detroit to pick up my parents from the airport. They never traveled light, so we parked the car and went inside to meet them at baggage claim. We waited so long that I spotted my mom's enormous flowered suitcase on the carousel before they got there. I had insisted that she get Dad a wheelchair at the airport, but when they showed up they were both walking. They had also obviously stopped for coffee on their way out. After hugging them I started in.

"Dad, why didn't you get a ride? This airport is huge!"

"Oh, he's fine," my mom answered for him. My dad shrugged and smiled.

"Happy Thanksgiving!" Kelsey said, hugging them both enthusiastically.

"How's my girl?" asked my dad. He always treated his grandkids as if they were the best children who ever lived, no questions asked.

"Where's my grandson?" said my mom, disapproval in her voice.

"We had to leave very early, Ma. You don't want to see Eliot when he's sleep deprived." She pursed her lips. "By the way, where are your masks? You know Covid is still going around, right?"

"Stop scolding, Jennifer Lynn, it's giving you wrinkles. We've had our vaccines, and anyway, the plane wasn't even full." *Okay, Boomer.* "Have you lost weight?"

This was her not-very-subtle way of remarking that I had, in fact, gained weight. I chose to ignore it.

"No, but thanks. Here, let us take those."

I grabbed my mom's huge suitcase and Kelsey took my dad's smaller one. He seemed a bit tentative on his feet so we walked very slowly to the car. My mom sat shotgun so Dad could sit in back with his adoring granddaughter. It didn't take long for me to regret having brought up masks.

"You know, my friend Lola from pickleball is a doctor," said my mother, before we were even out of the parking garage, "and she says she gave ivermectin to two people and it healed them! But her medical board won't allow her to prescribe it and she's really upset about it."

My eyes met Kelsey's in the rearview mirror.

"Isn't that horse de-wormer, Mom?" I asked.

"Yes, but it's used on humans sometimes."

"For parasites, though, right?"

"Lola's not stupid!" Mom protested, as if she'd been poised and ready to meet this resistance from her academic daughter. "She reads the medical journals."

"I'm sure she does, Mom, but..." I put my credit card in the machine, "*which* medical journals is she reading if she goes against her whole medical association?"

"Well which medical journals do YOU read?" she asked, leaning close to me, her eyes wide as if to say, *"Touche!"* I stared at her with my mouth hanging open till the person behind us honked. *Quick, change the subject.*

"Hey, speaking of horses," I drove on, "do you know what we learned this morning? Tell them, Kels, about the podcast we listened to." Her shell-shocked expression didn't change, but she took the hint.

"About anti-venom?" I nodded encouragingly. "Um, well, it was about how scientists make snake anti-venom by injecting venom into horses little by little, until their blood contains antibodies, because I guess horses' immune systems are kind of like human immune systems, and then they take the horses' blood and..."

"Oh, did you see that video," my mother interrupted, "of the snake in the Christmas tree?" Now Kelsey's mouth hung open. "This African family was just decorating their

Christmas tree and all of a sudden this snake came wandering out!"

She waved her right hand back and forth through the air like a snake puppet. The full cup of Starbucks decaf in her left waved and sloshed a little bit through the hole in the lid.

"You have to see it!" she exclaimed, "It's just so terrifying!" She handed Kelsey her phone. "Here, Google 'South African snake in a Christmas tree'."

We made it home around noon and I preheated the oven. Since there were so few of us, I had purchased a Tofurkey for my son and a chicken for the rest of us. I had bought pies and cranberry sauce from the Mennonites, and the night before I had slow-roasted a bunch of vegetables for re-heating.

While things were in the oven, the kids had a Zoom chat with their paternal grandparents, who were celebrating at Moose's brother's house. I had set up the Zoom for them on my computer ahead of time, but I didn't stay on much beyond 'Hello' and 'Happy Thanksgiving.' It was just too sad and awkward for me, and I suspected for them too. (I knew the kids would also talk to Moose sometime that day, but I didn't feel responsible for scheduling that.)

I left the kids in my office and went back to join my mom at the kitchen table while my dad dozed on the sofa.

"How are they?" my mother asked about my former in-laws. "We haven't seen them or talked to them since you left."

"As far as I know they're fine," I shrugged. "I haven't really talked to them either. I'll probably see them at Christmas."

"Are you divorced yet?" she asked.

"Marilyn," my dad warned from the other room. I guess he wasn't actually sleeping.

"Not yet. I called a lawyer and found out you have to be a Michigan resident for six months before you can get a divorce here. She suggested we figure some things out in the meantime so I downloaded some DIY divorce forms and Moose and I have been doing some unofficial negotiating."

"You talk to him?" she asked incredulously.

"Sometimes I have to, Mom. He's my kids' father. Anyway, it's fine. We're both behaving like adults. He's giving me the house and the minivan, and we agreed to split up all our joint accounts fifty-fifty except his 401K and my 403B. And he'll keep sending money for the kids as long as they're with me."

"But what about your future?" she asked hysterically. "And your kids' future? He's always made so much more money than you!" *Thanks for the reminder, Ma. As if I could forget.*

"That's where the lawyer will help us."

"You have to think about these things, Jennifer Lynn."

"Yes, I know, Mom," I raised my voice ever so slightly, "but I don't always have the energy to think about it between my job and dishes in the sink and a pile of laundry in the basement the size of K2!"

I got up from the table and went to the sink to wash said dishes.

"Give it a rest, Marilyn," my dad called in. It normally irked when my dad shooshed my mom, but at that moment I was grateful.

When the dinner hour arrived, we sat down in the actual dining room. It was normally reserved for piles of homework and reserve bags of cat food and litter, but Kelsey had made it lovely and festive. She had set the table with silverware and the good china – wedding gifts from way back. She had also assigned seats with homemade name tags on the plates, and had arranged tiny pumpkins and beeswax candles (also from the Mennonites' store) down the center of the table.

"What is that," my mother said pointing at the brown lump in front of Eliot.

"It's Tofurkey," he said. She looked horrified.

"This chicken looks delicious," my dad interjected.

"I hope so," I said. "It's Ina Garten's 'perfect roast chicken' recipe."

"Ina Garten?" Eliot said, almost smiling. "Does Jeffrey love it?" Kelsey laughed.

I was stunned. "You know Ina Garten and Jeffrey?"

Eliot said, "Yeah, well, there's just this guy on TikTok. 'Have you seen my husband, Jeffrey? I think he just went to my local fishmonger.'" He added a little chuckle, in a very good imitation of Ina Garten. (Or someone imitating Ina Garten.) "It's gonna be a great party. Yikes."

I had to hand it to the internet: my kids caught a lot of my generational references thanks to its depths.

Jamie had Thanksgiving dinner with her cousins, but she came over later in the evening for dessert. She arrived in a retro-looking orange overcoat, carrying a bag of supplies for making sober mocktails to go with the pie. I had tried to prepare my parents ahead of time so they wouldn't gawk, and they did pretty well, although even I sometimes still felt like gawking at Jamie. She was always such a sight to behold.

"It is so lovely to meet you both," she said. "Thank you so much for sending me your daughter and your grandkids."

"Well, we miss having them nearby," my mom said.
"I'm certain of that. I've only known them a couple of months and I would already be lost without them." She put her hand on Kelsey's shoulder and my daughter beamed. "Anyway it's wonderful that you could make it. And how are you feeling after your mishap?" She chatted with my dad while I hung up her coat and carried her supplies into the kitchen.

Once we were settled, we sat around for an hour or so eating pie, drinking warm pumpkin-spice digestifs ("Don't you diss the pumpkin spice," she had warned Eliot when he scoffed), and talking about St. Jutta. My dad was participating and smiling but I could tell he was exhausted, despite his nap.

"Do you need to go to bed, Dad?" I asked during a lull.

"I'm afraid I might, sweetheart." To Jamie he said, "I'm sorry to break up the party."

"Not at all! You've had a long day. I should be going anyway."

"It was very nice to meet you," he said. I motioned to Eliot to help his grandfather get off the sofa. He followed my dad slowly down the hall to the office-guestroom. The ladies chatted for a few minutes longer, slowly creeping toward the door in a bunch like an amoeba—the Midwestern goodbye.

"Thanks for making it a party," I said as I helped Jamie with her coat.

"Thanks for letting me meet the parents," she said, kissing me on the cheek. I felt a little flip just below my heart. *Pumpkin spice.*

"Now we're really friends," I laughed. "I'm sorry I never got to meet your parents."

"Me, too," she smiled. "They would have loved you."

I opened the door and basked in the cold air as she went out into the night. I always felt a little sad to see her leave.

Eliot hadn't returned yet, so I went to the office-guestroom. He and my dad were lying across the bed together, on their bellies and face to face, as if they had simply collapsed there. Four feet hung off the edge, and my son's arm was draped comfortingly over my dad's shoulder. Dad looked like a big, exhausted baby. I almost asked if he was okay, but hesitated because it seemed they were having a moment that shouldn't be interrupted. The scene was so touching that I felt myself about to cry.

Then my mom entered in business mode. "Come on, Bill, let's get ready for bed."

My dad groaned.

"Love you, Grandpa," Eliot said, slowly pushing himself up from the bed.

"I love you, grandson," my dad said, still prone.

"Oh, you're so sweet," my mother said suddenly, hugging Eliot around the waist. He hugged her back, almost as if he meant it.

The weeks between Thanksgiving and winter break were a whirlwind on campus. I was still recovering from four days with my parents. Students and faculty alike were emotionally done with their classes, but still had final projects and exams and grading ahead of them. Fran and I did our best to field all the crises that came through the door, one at a time. I told her our main goal—even when we couldn't fix things, which was usually—was to stay calm and not make anything worse.

Day after day I would send my kids off to school, Eliot masked and Kelsey unmasked (the schools seemed determined to make it all the way to the break in person, masks optional, despite several new cases every day). I kept doing this even after a shooting at Oxford High School a couple of hours away, letting them out of my sight as if they were unbreakable, as if I wouldn't be lost without them. Kelsey would always say goodbye and come in for a squeeze, but Eliot made me go to him, waiting dutifully by the door, his backpack in place as armor, for his enforced hug.

"I love you." I would say, always adding, "Be careful," as if these magic words could keep them safe. As if my warnings would be enough to prevent him from speeding or texting while driving, or to keep dangerous people away from my babies.

I suppose it was my secular version of a prayer.

Eliot would sigh and walk out the door without a word. He did pretty much the reverse upon returning home in the evenings, while Kelsey would regale me with the latest tales of middle school drama—who liked whom, who was mad at whom, who got in trouble, who smelled bad, who had the biggest boobs, who had the newest iPhone or Vans, who got the best grades. My mind reeled.

I didn't really love being in my fifties so far, but it sure as hell was better than being thirteen.

<Hey girlfriend, wanna do something fun tomorrow?> came a text on the first Friday in December.

<God yes. [anguished face]>

<Come with me to Lansing for a cheesy holiday parade and tree lighting! [snow person emoji] [Christmas tree emoji] Kids too!>

<OK! What time?>

<Leave at 5? I'll drive.>

<Awesome! Thank you so much! [pink hearts]>

"Isn't the Boy coming?" Jamie asked when we arrived on her doorstep. Eliot and Jamie were pretty tight by that time, thanks to regular running dates they'd started after cross country season ended.

"He briefly considered it—which is a huge compliment to you—but ultimately he declined when he realized he and Anna could have the house to themselves for a few hours."

"Ah, young love," she sighed.

In the car Kelsey sat shotgun, which was fine with me because it gave me the best chance to watch the two of them interact.

"What's the St. Judy Middle School goss this week?" Jamie asked. "Tell me absolutely everything."

"OMG," Kelsey obliged, "Ainsley and Trinity are in a huge fight over Connor T. because Ainsley has loved Connor T. for years and Trinity knows it, and then Trinity kissed Connor T. at Ashton's birthday party during spin the bottle last weekend!"

Kids still play spin the bottle?

"No!" Jamie shouted, eyes still on the road ahead.

"Yes!" Kelsey confirmed, eyes on Jamie, delighted to have found an eager audience.

"Ugh, middle school is the worst. That kind of happened to me once, only I was Ainsley, and Connor T. was played by Shelly, Queen of the Nerds, and my best friend Michelle kissed Shelly behind the port-o-potties at the softball field." Jamie held up one hand to her forehead and gasped dramatically. "Heartbreaking!"

"Awwwww, poor little Jamie," Kelsey said sympathetically.

"See, Kels?" I interjected. "Even Jamie struggled in middle school." *Would Jamie and I have been friends in middle school?*

"Meh," Jamie waved us off, "Shelly can eat her heart out. Tell me more!"

Kelsey continued to fill us in on the latest. Jamie ate it up, occasionally stopping to sing along with Ella Fitzgerald, who was singing holiday songs on the car stereo. We joined in too, letting it snow and having ourselves a merry little Christmas. My heart beat a little faster and my cheeks grew warm, but it didn't feel like a hot flash.

We parked and walked a few blocks, following the crowds flowing toward the capitol. At a street market, we bought fuzzy, glittery handmade hats with faux fur pompoms from a Detroit-based woman and her daughter, who knitted them by hand. We got some hot candied almonds in a paper bag from the next little tent and then went in search of hot chocolate. It was pleasantly cold and surprisingly crowded.

Lansing looked like an interesting place, and I made a mental note to visit more often. It was about seventy miles away, but that only took an hour from St. Jutta. It often took well over an hour to drive thirty miles from New Jersey to Manhattan and we used to do that several times a year, until Eliot learned about climate change and started making us take the train.

At the end of the night, the party planners lit up a giant tree on the capitol lawn and set off what I thought were fireworks, till they started turning into pictures and saying things like "Happy holidays" and "Peace on earth." They were drones, lighting up the sky.

Amid the blur of that first semester, the only times I really experienced the passing of time were during my short walks to and from work. The mornings and evenings gradually got darker, until I was both leaving the house and coming home to it in the dark. The plant life changed color, while my wardrobe choices grew thicker and more forgiving.

On the last day of finals week I had a lot of last-minute checklists to complete to make sure grading went smoothly for students and faculty and the registrar, and I had to pre-pare for the ever-growing slew of students suffering from anxiety and depression, who would inevitably be put on academic probation. I left home even earlier than usual, before the kids, so I could get some work done before other folks came in.

It was crazy windy outside, and yet freakishly warm. A neighbor's wind chime clanged in a minor key. The patch of pine trees on the corner swayed like an underwater crea-ture, and the naked branches on the oaks and maples waved vigorously as if in greeting (or perhaps warning, who could tell?). I half walked, half ran to the office, pushed by every gust. I felt like one of the leaves swirling and tumbling and spiraling down the middle of the empty street.

Most of the students had already gone home, and beyond the dragon gate threshold campus was eerily quiet. St. Mar-garet stood alone in on her pedestal, abandoned but solid in her equanimity, unflustered by the elements, her hooded face in shadow under the nearest light pole. Something in my chest wanted to stop and grieve—for my dad, for my kids, for my marriage, for the downfall of higher education, for the climate—right there in the quad. Margaret seemed to invite me to do so.

Stop it, Margaret. If I let myself think too hard I'll collapse, and I don't have time for that. People are depending on me. And besides, I really need to pee.

Chapter 13

Crappy Holidays

When the students were all gone but the grading was still under way, the president hosted his annual holiday party. Every employee was invited, except the catering staff who had to work it. (The COO reminded me they were outsourced and not technically college employees anyway.) Covid had put the kibosh on the holiday festivities in 2020, but this year—though Michigan was in and out of first place for "state in the US with the most cases"—Norm Festerling declared it was time to get back to normal.

"This is what our constituents want," he'd said. By "constituents" I had to assume he meant the most bro-ish members of the board of trustees and cabinet.

My constituents were just the opposite. Most of them were natural introverts, exhausted from being forced into small rooms with large groups of people day after day, and the last thing they wanted was to attend a supposedly festive, semi-obligatory gathering of a hundred unmasked (and probably several unvaxxed) people.

"Dear Dr. Smith-Miglione," wrote an assistant professor from the math department who was still too afraid to call me Jen, "I am writing regarding the president's party. I am pregnant as you know and my toddler is still too young for the vaccine. I don't feel comfortable being in crowds when there are so many cases of COVID-19 in our area. Do you think not going will reduce my chances of getting tenure? I asked my department chair and he told me to ask you. Thank you very much for your advice. Sincerely, Dr. Grace ----."

"Hi, Grace (if I may)," I wrote back, "I understand and share your concerns. I can assure you that your attendance at this or any other social gathering will have absolutely no bearing on tenure decisions. Your health comes first! And congratulations again on your pregnancy. Be well and happy holidays, Jen."

Another email came from the guy who hated administrators. "Jennifer," he wrote, "I am quite frankly astonished at the brazen and willful ignorance toward CDC and local health department recommendations that President Festerling's holiday party represents. I will not be attending this event, nor will I recommend that anyone of my acquaintance attend. It is quite frankly shameful that the administration is so wantonly playing fast and loose with the health of the College's employees, especially the faculty, without whom there would be no education of our students, by coercing people into attending what will almost certainly become a super-spreader event." He signed off with just his auto-signature.

I had to think for a few minutes about how best to respond to this one. *Quite frankly, dude, I can't imagine anyone asking you for social or health recommendations, and the party will be a lot better without you there. Stay home with my blessing.* He seemed mainly to be venting; I couldn't discern any actual questions or requests that needed action from me. And I more or less agreed with him, but he didn't need to know that. Then again, I also didn't feel the need to defend the president. I figured I'd basically reiterate what I'd told the math prof.

"Dear Geoffrey," I replied, "Thank you for sharing your concerns. I completely understand your decision to protect your health, and I assure you that there is absolutely no obligation to attend the president's party. Good luck with your grading and have a restful holiday break. Sincerely, Jen."

In hopes of preempting a slew of similar emails, I composed an email to the entire academic sector:

> Valued colleagues,
>
> Several of you have expressed understandable concern about attending President Festerling's holiday party this week. I want to assure you that attendance at this party is completely voluntary, rather than mandatory or even expected. Those who wish to attend are welcome to do so, but no one should feel at all compelled to go.
>
> Many of you know that, out of an abundance of caution, I have decided not to host the Provost's traditional academic sector holiday luncheon this year. Instead, Fran and I have prepared gift bags for each faculty and staff member in our sector. You are invited to stop by our office on Thursday or Friday of finals week to pick up these small tokens

of my esteem and appreciation for your hard
work during another difficult term.

I signed off "Warmest regards" because it reminded me
of *Schitt's Creek* and sometimes I needed a little private
joke to get me through the day.

Fran and I had purchased a variety of $20 gift cards to St.
Jutta businesses—Meijer (which also had a gas station), the
Dragon's Lair pub, Judy's Cafe, and of course Flyover Pride
Books. We laid these out on a table in the bay, along with
small brown gift bags and a selection of fresh masks, individually-wrapped snacks (*sorry, seventh generation*), and
mini-bottles of champagne or Pellegrino. They were able to
pack the bags themselves based on their tastes.

Fran surreptitiously checked takers off a list as they came
in and replenished the gift buffet as necessary. I lurked in
my office waiting for visitors. Having them stop by like this
gave me a chance to greet and thank lots of them personally, and even to meet a couple of the most reclusive ones
for the first time.

"This is such a lovely idea," said a biologist named Janine as she looked over the gift table, selecting a bag of
nuts and a book shop gift card. Janine could often be seen
knitting during faculty meetings, even on Zoom, and she
had reputedly been "about to retire" for at least a decade.
"The provost's luncheon is never very good for me anyway
because of my Celiac's. Ooo and I love champagne."

"I still think it's irresponsible for the president to host
a party," said Geoffrey under his mask. He hung back at a
distance while Janine made her selections. Begrudgingly he
added, "But yes, this was a nice idea, thank you." I counted
it a small win.

Those who never picked up their gift bags got one of the gift cards in their mailboxes. We also filled a few bags and left them for the staff who cleaned the academic buildings overnight. It wasn't perfect, but I hoped it at least sent the right signal.

The night of the president's party, I decided to put on a dress instead of my usual pantsuit. It seemed more festive, and I didn't want to look like someone's boss when people were supposed to be relaxing and having a good time.

Most of my dresses either didn't fit me anymore, thanks to my expanded midriff, or they were too low cut and "boobular," as my aunt liked to say, especially now that I kind of spilled out over most of my bras. I wistfully recalled the lost days of wishing for bigger boobs (*We must, we must, we must increase our bust!)* and made a mental note to order some new bras over the break. Meanwhile I opted for a low-cut, plum-colored dress that just barely still zipped and was dark enough that I could afford to risk a glass of red wine, which seemed like a provostly thing to drink. I planned to add a silk scarf to cover my fleshy cleavage.

Unfortunately, wearing a dress meant one thing: SPANX. I often wore some kind of lesser shapewear under my trousers, but SPANX were so extreme that I reserved them for only the most urgent situations.

I pulled a pair of full-length black hose from my underwear drawer and inspected them. I had a complicated love-hate relationship with SPANX. On one hand, they did indeed tighten up the parts of my body that embarrassed me the most, so I could spend less time worrying about what people might be thinking about my body. But wearing them also made me feel defeated and decidedly anti-feminist, for giving into the capitalist plot to get rich by shaming women into hiding their real bodies. (That SPANX were invented by a Gen X woman who was now a billionaire philanthropist only added to my ambivalence.)

But there was nothing for it if I was going to dress up in a professional setting. I sighed, peed one last time, and girded up my mental loins for the process of girding up my physical ones.

Getting into a pair of SPANX always involved some gymnastics. First I sat on the bed and pulled them over my feet and up to my ankles. I was already out of breath after leaning over for a few seconds, and that was the easy part. After that, I had to alternate between rolling back on the bed with my legs in the air, pulling downward on one leg at a time, and standing and/or jumping, pulling upward. I did this three or four times, and during what should have been my final, triumphant upward pull, I felt something snap in my neck. I swear I even heard a sound, like a rubber band launched from its maximum stretching point.

"Fuck!" I hollered, falling over onto the bed. My head was bent to the side and I couldn't move it.

"Mom!" Kelsey yelled from the doorway. "What are you doing in here? It sounds like an elephant stampede."

"I'm trying to get dressed and I hurt myself," I whined. She gaped at me in at my half-dressed state before she started giggling.

"It's not funny!" I said. My neck was killing me. Then I giggled too. "Ow, help me! I have to go to work."

She gently helped me stand up, and then put my dress down on the floor so I could step into it. She pulled it up and helped me get it on and then, with effort, zipped up the back while I held my breath.

"Thanks, hon," I said, seating myself on the bed. "Would you mind getting me some drugs from the bathroom?"

"Which ones?"

"Ibuprofen, please. Four of them," I added. She came back with the pills and some water and I swallowed them without moving my neck. I wanted to lie down for a minute but that seemed dangerous so I just kept sitting on the bed. Kelsey found my shoes and put them on the floor in front of me so I could squeeze my bloated feet in. I asked her to warm up my heating pad in the microwave while I put on my makeup.

When I got downstairs I poured myself a shot of tequila and drank it. Then I sat tentatively on a barstool and wrapped the pad around my neck. I would have given anything right then to put my pajamas on and stay home.

"Poor Ma," she said. "Is there anything else I can do before I go to Avery's?" (Trinity and her dad were soon coming to drive the girls to their postponed Halloween sleepover.)

"No thanks, hon, I really appreciate your help." I tried to smile but probably grimaced instead. "Actually, could you go get Eliot?"

When the kids came down, I asked him, "Could you please walk me over to the president's?"

His shoulders fell and his head bobbled backward.

"I'm sorry to ask, hon, but Kelsey's on her way out and it's dark and I'm afraid I might fall 'cause I can't really look down right now."

He whisper-groaned but went and got his coat. Kelsey got mine and carefully put it on me, even buttoning up the front, then retrieved my missing glove which Fiona had removed from the hallway to the living room. My daughter kissed me and I wished her a fun sleepover, before my son and I walked out into the night, my arm through his arm.

As we walked, I asked him how school was and he said "fine." I asked him how Anna was and he said "fine." I asked how his friends were and he said "I dunno."

Luckily it was a short walk.

The president's "mansion," a tall brick box with lots of windows (not much of a mansion by today's standards but probably impressive back in the day), looked cozy and inviting from the outside. It was decked from top to bottom in holiday lights.

"Thanks for getting me here safely, sweetie," I said to my firstborn. "I really appreciate it."

"Do I have to come back and get you?" He was already backing away before I had the chance to kiss him.

"No, thanks, I should be ok once the drugs kick in."

He scurried off and I carefully walked up the front steps, putting on my brave face as I opened the door and entered the foyer, where the president was greeting newcomers.

"Jennifer, welcome," he said formally. "Glad you could join us." It occurred to me that he was probably working from an administrator script, to stave off awkwardness, of the sort I myself was trying to develop.

"Hi, Norm, thanks so much for hosting." We shook hands. The redheaded woman from the giant portrait on his office wall stood stiffly just behind him. She was a few years older but perfectly coiffed, tastefully dressed in a forest green, short-sleeved sheath dress that only a thin person could get away with. Her orange mane cascaded sleekly over her shoulders. In her heels she was almost as tall as Norm. She looked like Princess Fiona in human form, while I was the ogress version.

"I don't believe you've met my wife, Helen?" The princess extended her hand. *Back to normal.* I would have to remember not to touch my face till I could give my hands a good scrubbing when this was all over. "Jennifer is just finishing up her first semester as provost."

"Oh, right," she said, the lights going on. I wondered what he'd already told her about me, if anything. "Nice to meet you, Jennifer."

"So nice to meet you, too, Helen. Thank you for having us. It looks lovely in here." It smelled good too, like baking butter, and maybe mushrooms. The sound of subdued merriment echoed from the next room.

"Yes, well it's our pleasure." She must have had an administrator's wife script. "May I take your coat?"

Gingerly I disrobed in front of my boss and his wife, trying not to move my neck. While she hung up my coat in a closet, I was horrified to realize in the bright light of the chandelier that, in all the commotion at home, I had forgotten my scarf. This meant my cleavage was on full display. Thankfully the tequila was kicking in.

"Have a good time," Norm said, tactfully not looking at my chest. I thanked them one more time, straightened my posture as well as I could, and strode confidently into the living room.

It was as kitchily festive as a Christmas card, with evergreen trim and fake candles and red bows. A giant tree, elegantly decorated with only maroon and gold ornaments, stood in one corner. My old boss in New Jersey had always been careful to honor diversity around this time of year, making sure there were a variety of religious and traditional symbols, with Diwali lanterns and menorahs and Dongzhi dumplings interspersed among the greenery and frosted cookies. No such effort had been made here. Rural Michigan really was a different world. *It is a Catholic school, Jen. What did you expect?*

I was already starting to sweat through my dress. For a second I felt envious of the kitchen workers, who got to wear sneakers and black cotton shirts and pants, and who had trays to carry and a kitchen to hide in. *Come on, Jen, you're a professional so start acting like it.* I began making my rounds, trying to talk to as many people as I could without turning my neck. I sometimes had to turn my whole body toward someone if they came at me from behind or from the side. I hoped it wasn't too noticeable.

"Are you ok?" asked the orchestra director when I turned to greet him.

I guess it was noticeable.

"Oh, yeah," I laughed, trying to sound casual, "just pulled my neck a little bit getting...doing yard work." He looked puzzled at the mention of yard work in December but let it go. The art professor standing next to him, Brittany, chimed in.

"Oh no!" she said sympathetically. "I pull things all the time now. It's like somebody flipped a switch when I turned 40 and everything just started breaking. Planned obsolescence or something like that." It was nice of her to share but it also freaked me out a little, because she looked a lot older than 40 to me. How old must I look, especially with a broken neck?

"I'm going to go get some wine," I said. "Do you want anything?"

On the way to the bar I saw Fran standing near the tree with her husband, eating hors-d'oeuvres off a real plate. They both held glasses of water.

"Hello there," I said a tad awkwardly. Fran gave me a tepid nod. Jason's expression was friendly but blank. "It's good to see you again, Jason. I'm Jen. We met on Opening Day."

"Oh, yeah," he smiled with sudden recognition, "I can even shake your hand now that I'm not covered in blood."

"Dear!" Fran looked embarrassed. I took his hand and laughed to set her at ease.

"Did you catch anything?" *Obviously, Jen, unless the blood was human.*

"Yes, ma'am, we sure did. Got a big eight-point buck."

"Wow." I assumed that was good. I was totally out of hunting questions. "Do you all have plans for the break?"

"Nothing too big," he said cheerfully. "Our kids'll come home for a few days and we'll get together with my family on Christmas eve and her family on Christmas day."

"That sounds nice." No further information was forth-coming. I wanted a drink and didn't have the energy to try to woo Fran tonight. "I hope you all have a great time. Can you point me toward the bar?"

I finally made it to the bar, where a young man who could have been a student, but wasn't, poured me a huge glass of mediocre cabernet. I thanked him and gulped half of it before turning away. Thus fortified, I continued work-ing the room, remembering not to slouch.

I stopped in with the Xennial scientists' clique, where they were talking about the new *Matrix* reboot. I hadn't seen it, but had re-watched the trilogy with Eliot during early Covid, so I was at least somewhat literate. I moved on to a clique of young women, a mix of untenured and non-tenure-track instructors, where they were discussing their CrossFit regimes. They looked anxious to have me there, so I offered some stupid joke about never exercising and headed over to the old dudes' clique.

"Gentlemen," I greeted them.

"Well, hello there, young lady," said a jolly accountant named John. I wondered if he'd worked with Jamie's dad. "Nice dress." He looked at my chest. I stood up straighter.

"It's good to see you all."

"I never miss free food and drink on the administration's dime," said a normally quiet painter named Sam. "It's one of the few perks left about working here." He had apparently partaken of enough beer to loosen his lips.

I didn't want to let that go by without comment. "Has it been a hard semester?"

"Hard semester, hard decade." He shook his head.

These guys had entered higher ed in the good old days when there were plenty of students and plenty of funding, and not enough professors to go around. They didn't all have PhD's, hadn't published anything scholarly or taught a new class for years, and wanted to retire but couldn't afford to. Still, they somehow managed to terrorize all their younger, much better-qualified colleagues.

"Things are nothing like they used to be," he said, "and this administration has no idea what they're doing. No offense."

"None taken." *You're the provost for all of them, and he's not wrong.* "I know things have been really hard since 2008, especially in the arts and humanities." My glass was almost empty and I longed for another. We were rescued from the litany of academia's woes when the president called for a toast.

"If I could have your attention everyone," Norm said blandly, "Helen and I would like to thank you all for coming to this beautiful event. It's been a challenging semester for all of us..." (at that point an unintentionally-audible "Ha!" escaped me and he glanced at me briefly before going on) "...but you've made it through with flying colors, and I am so grateful for everything you do for the College of St. Margaret." (He never called it St. Margaret's because the branding team had said it was important to always use its proper name.) "Wish you all a wonderful holiday and let's have a toast to the new year."

I noticed he didn't have a drink and wasn't actually joining in his own toast. *That's a real power move*, I thought. *Everyone else is getting sloshed and stuffed and he walks around like, like...* I couldn't think of an appropriate simile. *This better be your last drink, Jen.*

"Hi, Jennifer," someone behind me said. It was Vivian, the dance professor. I had given up on people calling me Jen here; it was apparently too informal for a provost. They seemed more comfortable keeping me at arm's length. I turned my whole body around.

"Oh hi, Vivian!" I said too cheerfully. She gave me the up and down—or what the kids called elevator eyes.

"That's a flattering dress." I thanked her, even though it was obvious that "flattering" held a covert insult from someone who was 5'10" and a size 2 and had never once had to worry about her clothes being flattering. Absolutely everything looked amazing on her, even at her age, which I guessed was somewhere in her early-to-mid-60s.

"What are your plans for the holidays?" I asked, changing the subject.

"My daughter and granddaughter are coming for a visit from Florida. I'm hoping for snow; my granddaughter loves to go sledding if she can." I tried to imagine Vivian sledding.

"That sounds fun," I said. "How old is she?"

"Eleven," Vivian said.

"Oh, it's too bad we won't be home. I'm sure my daughter would love to meet her." I immediately regretted this comment. It sounded desperate. She politely ignored it.

"Where are you headed?" she asked.

"My kids and I are going to see my parents in New Jersey, and then they're going to visit their father and his family." That was probably more information than she wanted. I didn't know if Vivian was divorced or widowed or never married.

"Well that sounds lovely." She was done with me. "Have a merry Christmas."

"You too."

Most of the faculty left after the toast. By then my head was a little fuzzy and my feet hurt. I returned to the bar for a glass of ice water and then sat down in a wingback chair by the fireplace, till I thought better of it and moved to a less comfortable but cooler chair across the room. The young VP of admissions and one of her even younger minions were talking on the sofa, looking grave.

"Hi ladies, it's nice to see you." I tried to turn my chair toward them without being too obvious. "How are things over in your office?"

"Welllll," the VP hesitated, looking at her colleague. She always put a positive spin on things at cabinet meetings but I suspected she, too, had had a drink or two and might be more forthcoming. "Things really aren't looking too good," she admitted. "Our applications are way down across the board, both FTIAC and transfer students, and of course international students."

"What's fittiack?" asked the COO, suddenly standing over us. The enrollment VP stiffened. I suspected that she lived in fear of him firing her, as I had heard he'd been known to do without warning. The last enrollment VP had been called into his office one morning for a meeting and then escorted off campus immediately by campus security.

"First time in any college," I answered curtly. I felt annoyed at him for interrupting, for standing over us, and for still not having learned basic higher ed lingo. I gave him the side-eye (only partly because of my neck) and turned my attention back to the VP.

"You all have done an amazing job keeping our admissions numbers as high as they are." These numbers had of course come with increased numbers of drop-outs, but that wasn't entirely their fault; colleges everywhere were struggling to keep students. We'd struggled at Madison too, but Michigan was a whole different ball game—much poorer and less populous than the Northeast. Michigan's population had been shrinking for years, losing members of Congress with every census. The few remaining teenagers almost always picked a bigger state school in a cooler city—Grand Rapids, Ann Arbor, East Lansing, Detroit, Marquette—over tiny schools in sleepy towns in the flattest parts of the lower peninsula. "Admissions definitely has the hardest job of all," I said, which actually made me tear up a little. *Get a grip on yourself.*

"Thanks," they both said.

"A business can't survive without customers," the COO said. *Dude, get a new song.* The younger women looked at me beseechingly.

"We're all painfully aware of that." I was getting hot. I stood up so I could face him directly. "But their team has worked tirelessly to make sure the rest of us can keep going, and tonight is a night to celebrate their efforts." I turned back toward the couch and held up my water glass. "I salute you both!" I tried to drink the last drop but it hurt my neck. The COO walked away.

"Welp, I think my job is done here." The admissions people laughed tentatively. "Have a good night."

After a night of polite conversation in uncomfortable clothes, I was exhausted and nearly desperate for more pain medicine. Besides my neck, my feet hurt and my midriff pinched. I stopped by to thank Norm and Helen again for the evening, grabbed my coat from the front hall closet, and stepped out into the night before putting it on. The cold felt good on my bare decolletage. I could see peripherally that the sky was bright with stars, but between my neck spasm and my fear of falling I couldn't properly look up at them. I put on my coat without buttoning it and walked home.

My first stop inside was the kitchen for another shot of tequila, and then I headed upstairs to the medicine cabinet. I got four more ibuprofen, hoping my liver would tolerate this short-term extravagance. I kicked off my shoes and let my coat drop to the floor. I cursed silently upon realizing that I would need help unzipping my dress and Kelsey wasn't home, but my bladder was screaming at me so I first had to get out of my SPANX.

The next moments of my life happened in slow motion. I managed to pull up my dress without looking down, and I got my undergarment down past my butt. But as I tried to sit down on the bed to pull them off my legs, I missed and toppled sideways. I saw the corner of my dresser coming toward me, powerless to stop it. I think I hollered just before my face crashed into it, making a terrible noise. I lay on the floor for a few moments, stunned. When I stopped seeing stars, I looked up and beheld my son. He was beholding his prone mother—skirt around my waist, girdle of death around my knees, pubes and butt cheeks on full display. The look of horror on his face would give me nightmares for weeks.

"Hi, hon," I said, trying to sound casual while lying on the floor.

"Oh my god," he leaned over, "you're bleeding!"

"Um, could you get me a towel maybe?" He ran to the bathroom and came back with a white hand towel, putting it up to my face.

"Are you ok?"

"I'm fine," I laughed, "I'm just a klutz."

"No, Mom, it looks really bad." I was alarmed because he almost never called me Mom. I looked down at the towel and saw a shockingly red spot. *I'll need to soak that in cold water.*

"Can you bring me a darker towel?"

"Mom, seriously," he said, "it's bad. Your lip is like, ripped." I dabbed at my face again, a huge Rorschach blotch forming. I felt something wet on my eyebrow. "You also hit your forehead." He left and came back with another towel and held it to my head. With effort I pushed myself up, half lying, half sitting, like some pathetic mermaid, my neck still bent to one side. *God dammit, Moose, I could really use another adult right about now.*

"Well, shit." I looked him in the eye. "Son, I'm gonna need your help and it's not gonna be pretty."

Without a word, he got me seated on the bed and helped me take off the offending SPANX, followed by my dress. Wearing only my bra, and still holding two towels to my face, I limped into the bathroom to pee by myself while he picked me out some normal clothes. After helping me get those on, he held my coat around my shoulders, trying to maintain pressure on a towel while I put first one arm, then the other into the sleeves. He ran downstairs to warm up the car. I followed slowly. At the bottom of the stairs I slipped my bare feet into my boots, not bothering to zip them up. By the time I had those on he came back into the house to get me, closed the door behind us, helped me down the stairs and into the car. Still silent, he drove us to the ER.

Inside, I presented myself at the desk. "Hi there, I think I might need stitches." The waiting room was playing cheesy-ass, Kenny G-style Christmas music.

"Oh?" She looked bored. I removed the towel so she could see. "Oh, my goodness!" She suddenly seemed engaged and looked suspiciously at the tall, surly young man standing behind me.

"I fell down while I was trying to get out of my SPANX after a party," I explained.

"Ohhhh." She nodded in understanding. Eliot was off the hook. He sat in the waiting room for the next couple of hours while I got five stitches in my lip and two on my forehead.

It was after 1:00 a.m. when we got home. Eliot put my heating pad in the microwave while I went upstairs. In the bathroom mirror I saw a bruised, puffy face that I barely recognized. I half-heartedly brushed my teeth and took one of the heavy-duty painkillers they'd given me at the ER. I groaned as I crawled into bed, trying to make micro-movements that wouldn't jar my neck, or my head, or my face, or my fragile state of mind. When I finally stilled myself, the solidness of the mattress holding me securely, I sighed with relief.

Eliot came in with the heating pad. For a split second I could see him as his little boy self, a timid but cheerful kid who used to play with trains and make his own costumes out of construction paper. He now wore the expression of a rabbit about to dart into hiding. Poor guy. My overgrown bush was no doubt burned onto his traumatized brain forever.

He helped me arrange the heating pad under my neck and pulled his own weighted blanket over me. "Um, are you gonna be ok?"

At the sound of his manly voice my eyes welled up. "Yes, hon, I'm ok. I'm so sorry for all this. Thank you so much."

"OK, good night." He patted me on the head and scurried away, turning off the lights and closing the door on his way out. A faint sliver of light from the neighbors' back porch shone across the ceiling.

Alone in my bed, heat radiating up through my neck, blanket heavy on my torso, I started crying. I wanted to stop because it hurt to move and there were no tissues nearby, but it couldn't be helped. All the tensions and humiliations of the night—or maybe of the semester—came pouring out of me in a stream of tears and snot, making my head throb and my lip sting. I cried until I couldn't anymore, felt the salty goo turn crusty on my face, and somehow succumbed to sleep.

Chapter 14

Christmas in NJ

The day before the kids and I were scheduled to leave for New Jersey, I planned to work from home. I did not plan to receive an early morning email from a young faculty member in chemistry telling me he was quitting, effective immediately, for "personal reasons." *Fucking millennials*, was my first thought before correcting myself. *Your millennials are some of your most dedicated faculty members.*

I stared out the window for a minute, letting it sink in that I had to figure out what to do with three big classes, in one of our biggest majors, now in need of qualified instructors who had to be found and contracted during a holiday break. He had cc'd his department chair, so there was a panicked email from her as well. I spent the next hour in my sweats on Zoom with Ashley, the department chair, calming her fears.

"What would you *like* to do?" I asked her. She stared back anxiously. "I mean it—if you had total freedom to choose, what would you like to do about next semester?"

She thought for a few moments. "I don't know, I guess...maybe cancel his classes?" She seemed to scare herself with that suggestion and quickly added, "But of course I can teach his classes myself if we need it!"

I took a deep breath and tried to translate. "I think your first wish to cancel them all mostly means that you don't want to have to teach all of his classes yourself, and you're also not excited about trying to find folks to teach them on short notice. Is that a fair representation?" She hesitated.

"Yes, that's fair."

"Ok," I said, "we can work with that. I feel the same way. I don't think it would be a good idea to cancel *all* of his classes, but I also don't want you teaching them all. Let's figure out which ones we can do without and which ones we can't, and then I'll help you find someone to teach the ones we absolutely need. Sound good?" The relief on her face was palpable. Reminding her that there were other options was calming for me too.

"Yes, thank you so much," she said. "I was terrified that I was going to have to deal with this all by myself."

"Listen, you don't get paid enough, or have enough power, to have to deal with this kind of thing," I said. "This is a provost problem. That's why they pay me the big bucks." We both laughed.

"By the way," she asked, emboldened by my informality, "are you ok?" She gestured toward her forehead, reminding me of my fresh battle scars.

"Oh, ha, yeah." My hand automatically went to my face. "Long story. I'm fine, I'm just a klutz. I need to do Pilates or something." I wanted to change the subject before oversharing. "Out of curiosity, do you have any idea why he quit so suddenly? I know he's had a few hiccups along the way but this took me by surprise."

"Well, his wife just got a full-time law job in Chicago. I know they had been talking about living long distance, but I think the baby makes that untenable."

"I can certainly understand that," I sighed. "I just wish he'd given us a little heads up."

"Maybe he was afraid he'd get fired before he was ready to leave?"

"Yeah." I nodded. "He obviously failed to consider what a monumental pain it is to try to hire a new faculty member, right?"

We talked about options and ultimately decided I would ask the other faculty members in the department if they wanted to pick up an extra class, prioritizing those that upper-class majors needed before graduation. After seeing how many were left unclaimed, we'd decide what to cancel and to fill some other way. When we hung up I crafted an email to the rest of the department (chemistry was one of our largest, thanks to all the students laser-focused on getting into med school or nursing or other health careers). I summarized the situation, letting them know they were neither required nor expected to take on another course at such short notice, but to let me know if they wanted one before I started looking for adjuncts.

Then I replied to the faculty member who had quit (cc-ing HR), accepting his resignation and telling him I would follow up after the holidays to see if we could talk about his decision. I also did a little research on what kinds of online, asynchronous course options we could buy for our students from another institution as a last resort.

At 9:32 I had a headache and realized I hadn't had any coffee yet so I went to make some. By the time I got back to my computer there were already replies from two chemistry professors, one who wanted an extra course, one who didn't. I let out a sigh. The situation was indeed a major inconvenience, but not a catastrophe. We'd manage with minimal pain to students and faculty.

It also brought about a lightbulb moment for me. We spent a lot of money on adjuncts and overloads classes that weren't full or actually necessary to our students—money that could possibly go toward salary increases. I sighed again. *Now you really sound like an administrator.*

We flew to New Jersey on December 23rd, leaving for the airport in the wee hours. I drove and the kids mostly slept, giving me two hours to drink coffee and listen to the news and ruminate over all the end-of-semester meetings (with of course a stop to pee at some gas station in the middle).

I had gotten my stitches taken out by a PA at urgent care the night before—a day earlier than the ER doctor had recommended, but because of the holiday I had prevailed upon her to make an exception. The cuts themselves were pretty well healed, but there was still a greenish-yellow egg on my forehead (which I covered with a St. Margaret's beanie) and a huge purple scar and bruise on my lip. I had warned my parents with a photo the night before we left, which Jamie and Kelsey had helped me compose for optimum flattery and minimum shock.

"Are you sure you want pictures, Mom? You look terrible," Kelsey had said.

"I am aware, Kelsey. That's why I need to warn my parents."

"Nonsense!" Jamie had said. "She looks like a beautiful but tragic heroine with a dark secret. And really, isn't that the truth?" She kissed me on the unbruised side of my face before pulling Kelsey in for a hug. "I'm gonna miss you all so much!"

"We'll miss you too." I felt a little teary. I didn't want to pack my suitcase or get on an airplane. I wanted to stay home and snuggle with these two.

"What are you doing for Christmas?" Kelsey asked.

"I'm working at the store on Christmas eve and Boxing Day so I can sell as much merch as possible and my employees can have some time off. And on Christmas I'm sleeping late, taking a long bath, and then Deirdre and I are going on a road trip to Grand Rapids for Chinese food with my high school friend Asher and his family."

"Chinese food?"

"It's a Jewish tradition."

"You had a Jewish friend in St. Jutta?" I was genuinely surprised and asked without thinking. Luckily Jamie was Jamie.

"Well, Asher wasn't always Asher and wasn't always Jewish. That happened in our late twenties. It's a long story I'll tell you sometime. But right now you ladies need to get packed. It looks like you haven't even started!"

When we arrived in long-term parking at Detroit Metro it was still dark outside, but inside, the terminal was shiny and noisy and bustling with travelers. At my insistence we had only carry-ons so we headed straight to security, where there was a long snake of passengers waiting for the privilege of undressing and being x-rayed and yelled at like naughty children.

"This airport is a lot nicer than the one I grew up with," I said. "Newark is famously awful. Although it's being renovated now." Kelsey nodded. I had told them both they couldn't wear their earbuds till we were through security.

Eliot said, "Can we agree right now that you will spare us your back-in-the-day stories for the rest of the week?" A hot wave of petulance passed through me.

"Just for that," I responded, "I'm gonna tell you even *more* back-in-the-day stories. Like about the time I puked into a garbage can in Newark airport, right before saying goodbye to my Italian boyfriend the last time I ever saw him." He groaned and looked back at his phone.

"You had an Italian boyfriend?" Kelsey asked, astonished. I laughed out loud. *Thank you, God, for giving me a daughter.* Then, just in case anyone was actually listening, I added, *Sorry, I know that's gender essentialist.*

Our flight was mercifully uneventful; no one refused to wear a mask or assaulted a flight attendant. Despite exorbitant prices due to under-supply, I rented a car to spare my parents the spaghetti of ramps and frontage roads and Mad Max drivers around Newark airport. Having my own wheels would have the added benefit of guarding against me feeling trapped in my childhood home.

We headed west till we exited onto a small, curving highway that wound through a string of small historic towns, packed close together, full of tall trees and colonial architecture and schools named after founding fathers. It all screamed "George Washington slept here," so different from the sparsely-populated farmland grids of lower Michigan. I had the strange mix of feelings that comes from being somewhere familiar yet also from a distant memory, kind of like in dreams where you both do and don't know where you are. I must have been daydreaming at one of the many intersections because someone behind me blared his horn to let me know the light was green.

"That's where Brian Kennedy asked me to my first homecoming dance," I said as we drove on, pointing out the football field where we had marching band practice. "And that's where I used to go watch Josh Weitzman play goalie on the soccer team. Ooo, and that's where I had my first kiss with Joey LaRusso," I said, pointing out a tiny cemetery. *It was a terrible kiss but whatever.*

"Gosh, were you just boy crazy?" Kelsey asked.

"I dunno, maybe a little bit," I said. I thought about it. I suppose I was always fairly concerned about liking and being liked by boys, but wasn't everyone at that age? "A normal amount, I think."

"Ugh, I'm never gonna be like that," my daughter said. *From your lips to God's ears.*

We arrived at the house where I grew up, a white, colonial-style ranch with a low, mostly symbolic fence around my mother's dormant rose bushes. It looked exactly as it always did, except for the outdoor holiday lights, professionally done. We let ourselves in the front door.

"Mom, Dad, I'm home!" I said, like a kid on 70s TV.

"Well, great!" I heard my dad's voice from down the hall. We passed the living room where no one sat and walked into the den, where he was slowly on his way to greet us, looking a hundred percent better than at Thanksgiving, almost like his old self. "Hiya, sweetie!" He gave me a big hug.

"You look great, Dad!"

"Well, I feel great. You look great too." He winked.

"I do not, but thanks."

"Well you're a sight for my sore eyes, anyway. Hey, you kids, come here and give your Gramps a hug." They happily did as commanded. By then my mom had joined us and immediately started in.

"Jennifer Lynn! If I didn't know better I'd think you'd gotten into a fight!"

"I know, Mom, but I'm fine."

"I have some cream for that from my homeopath. She swears it can get rid of any scar!"

Dad saved me. "Come on in, take a load off. You want some coffee?"

I had peed at the airport but needed to go again. (I had even purchased some special pee-proof underwear on the web before we left, so paranoid was I about accidents.) "Yeah, just let us get our stuff out of the front hall."

This was the first time we had all stayed here as a family. The kids had occasionally had sleepovers with Gran and Gramps, but because we'd always lived close by, I hadn't slept here in decades. Eliot took his things into the guest room, and Kelsey and I took ours upstairs to my childhood bedroom. I dropped my bags in the hall and stepped into the bathroom, the same mauve and hunter green it had been since they'd had it redone in my youth. Sitting on the toilet, I texted Jamie.

<Kill me now! [xx-eye emoji]>

<No way! I would miss you too much!> she texted back.

When I got to the bedroom, Kelsey was arranging her things. I had dozed for a few minutes on the plane but my body felt heavy and sleepy. The bed—painted white with gold trim, circa 1984 and covered with a "dusty rose" bedspread—beckoned me to lie down, but my mom had pulled together a spread of sandwiches and snacks in the kitchen so I headed back downstairs.

Eliot, who was putting together a meat-free plate for himself, looked askance at me as I brewed a cup of coffee from the earth-destroying Keurig.

"I'm tired," I whispered. He shook his head. *Gimme this one thing, kid.*

It was going to be a long week.

On Christmas Eve we heard the news that a thousand U.S. flights had been canceled because too many airline workers were infected with Covid. My immediate reaction was to feel jealous of the passengers who got to stay home. Then I shamed myself for being ungrateful about getting to be with family for Christmas, especially the first year after my kids' father disappeared from their lives. And *then* my stomach lurched when I realized what this might mean for his flight from Costa Rica tomorrow. I desperately didn't want to see Moose, but I also desperately wanted my kids to have the chance to see him. I could tell they were both ambivalent about it—almost excited, but not quite—and I thought it was important for them to get that first-meeting-after-he-left-us out of the way.

That day we all went to lunch with my aunt and uncle, despite the germy throng. We planned to meet them at our favorite classic diner, Papa Guy's, which had a gigantic menu and served breakfast all day. When we arrived at 11:00 a.m. they were standing on the sidewalk waiting for us, holding hands and bundled up against the cold, my uncle in his tweed newsman cap and my aunt wrapped in a long wool coat topped with a purple crocheted shawl. They looked tiny and elderly, which made me feel a bit weepy.

This aunt and uncle were from the Italian side of my family—my mom's younger sister and her husband. I'd always been close to them. They were intellectuals, both Rutgers professors, and kind of the opposite of my mom and dad. They had provided an alternative vision of adult life while I was growing up. They never had kids—I wasn't sure if that was by choice or luck—and always lived in a funky two-bedroom apartment in New Brunswick, in a neighborhood that had once been gritty but was now firmly gentrified, to their chagrin. Where my parents were traditional, they seemed edgy and cool.

I swallowed hard and we all hugged and said our hellos, awkward in our human sidewalk amoeba, and I went inside to ask if they could manage a table for seven.

"Good morning," I said to the host upon entry, "how are you?"

"Living the dream," he said. I recognized him as the grandson of Papa Guy, who had grown significantly since I'd seen him last. (*Was that only last summer?*) He was an outgoing, dark-haired, refrigerator of a man, a bit older than Eliot, wearing a Santa hat and Christmas shirt. It slowly dawned on me that the shirt was actually a *trompe l'oeil* of a naked, hairy, muscle-bound chest with tree ornaments for nipple rings.

"Wow!" I said.

"Thanks," he said through a broad smile. "I like to watch people's faces as they try to figure out what's happening here." His hands gestured over his fake hairy chest. I wondered if such a shirt could survive a Title IX case. I hoped I'd never find out.

It was on the early side for lunch so there was plenty of room. Frank showed us to our table, handed out laminated menus, and said our waiter would be right with us. The waiter was similar in age but otherwise the opposite of Frank—a long, wiry ginger with a wispy beard and an overly cheerful manner. He had green fingernails and forearm tattoos and snapped his fingers every time he took an order. "Coffee?" (Snap.) "Absolutely!" "French fries?" (Snap.) "You got it!"

Later, when he put my food down in front of me, I noticed several thick lines, old scars, scratched across his pale skin amid his forearm tattoos. *Poor guy*, I thought. He was probably an extreme introvert whose abundance of cheerfulness and snapping were a script he used to cover up deep anxiety and existential sadness. I wanted to give him a motherly hug. *You're doing great, kid, keep it up.*

"Well how's life in the Motor City?" asked my uncle. To most people in New Jersey, even the smart ones, all of Michigan is Detroit.

"We are nowhere near the Motor City," I laughed, "we're in the farmland, but I think we're doing ok, right guys?" I looked toward my kids, hoping they might join in, but they both nodded half-heartedly.

"I still cannot believe you actually chose to move out there," said my aunt. "Isn't it basically Trump country?"

Even now, well into their 70s, there were still stark differences between her and my mom. My aunt let her facial hair grow free, and gray hairs mixed wantonly with her long, shaggy mop. She also had the round body of a stereotypical Italian *nonna*. My mother, on the other hand, did her best to embody the WASP ideal. She got her face waxed and her hair dyed every three weeks, went to Curves almost daily, and survived mainly on meat, white wine, and supplements.

Though she was the elder, she prided herself on looking much younger.

"I can't believe it either," she interjected. I guess they shared some qualities.

Before I could answer, I was saved by the server. My mother had ordered three different appetizers "for the table." We passed them around and welcomed the conversation they enabled. Eliot refused them all, but Kelsey dutifully tasted calamari, lamb bites, and escargots.

"Why aren't you eating, Eliot?" my mother asked him loudly.

"I only eat plant-based foods," he mumbled into his empty plate. I cringed. His voice was so low there was no way she had heard him.

"What?" she shouted, leaning in. I patted her lightly on the arm.

"I only eat plant-based foods," he said, slightly more loudly, and slightly in her direction. Kelsey, still chewing, took some more calamari.

"Are you a *vegan*?" my mother asked. It was obviously an accusation. *Are you now or have you ever been...*

"I just don't eat animals or animal products because it's better for them and the environment." He looked as if he wanted to sink into the ground.

"Well, I wish I had known that before," she protested. "We're having a roast tomorrow."

"Oh my god, Mare," my aunt said, "you sound just like Mama." That, coming from my aunt, was not a compliment. (Despite looking just like my Nonna, she had always been the *pecora nera* of the family.)

"It's fine, Mom," I said, patting her again and trying to defuse the situation. Then I felt bad about shushing her so

I put my hands back in my lap. "Eliot's a big boy. I promise he'll find enough to eat. He's survived the last four months in a house with me, right?"

My mom, rejecting the lifeline I was trying to throw her, shook her head and kept going. "I just hope he's getting enough protein. He's still growing, you know."

"Marilyn, take a breath." This was my dad, who hadn't said two words yet. "Everyone's telling you it's fine."

"These poor kids have to deal with so much," she sighed. "First their deadbeat father and now..."

"Mom!" I said sharply.

"Jesus, Mare!" shouted my aunt.

"Marilyn!" said my dad at the same time.

She finally seemed to get the message and went back to picking at her food. Eliot looked around the restaurant, presumably for the nearest escape route, and Kelsey looked at me as if she'd been slapped. I made a sympathetic face and mouthed, "Sorry." I was suddenly boiling hot and thought I might punch my mother if I didn't get my clothes off immediately. I began removing my sweater as elegantly as I possibly could, given the tight space. My dad noticed.

"Uh oh," he said quietly, "are you going through 'the change'?"

"Yup," I laughed. "How does it feel, Dad, to have a daughter who gets hot flashes?"

Without missing a beat he replied, "How does it feel to have a dad who wears diapers?" I was stunned for half a second and then we both cracked up.

"What?" my mother asked.

"Nothing," I said. My dad winked at me.

Later that night, as Kelsey and I snuggled into my childhood bed, she asked, "Why did Gran call Dad a deadbeat?"

"Oh hon," I said, "I'm sorry about that. She's just angry at him for leaving us. For leaving *me*, I mean. I'm still her little girl."

"Would you be mad if my husband left me?"

"Of course!" I said. "I love you more than anything in the world, so I'm automatically angry at anyone who hurts you." I kissed her forehead and turned out the light. We lay quietly in the dark for a moment, till she spoke again.

"Dad hurt you?"

I paused to formulate an appropriate answer. I had been trying so hard not to put my baggage on my kids, but I also didn't want to lie to her.

"Yes," I finally said. "It hurt me a lot that he left." There was a lump in my throat so I took a deep breath and stopped there.

"Aw, I'm sorry, Mom." She rolled over, put her head on my shoulder, and stretched her arm around me. "All this time I thought you were fine."

Chapter 15

Dead Week

Christmas morning was pretty relaxed. I had bought bagels the day before—real, toothy bagels from a deli, not that spongey supermarket nonsense—and we gorged ourselves on them with lox and cream cheese (or in Eliot's case, a slice of tomato and capers) in between opening stockings and presents. My mom couldn't resist playing Santa Claus every year, so she bought way too many gifts for everyone and the living room looked like a department store display. I sighed, thinking about having to get to the post office to ship all that stuff home before we left.

Traditionally I had always brought little things to fill my parents' stockings but I had totally forgotten this year. I kicked myself for the deflated socks hanging forlorn from the mantle. I made a mental note to do something nice for them while I was here. I knew us leaving hadn't been easy on them, and they deserved a daughter who was fully present when I was around.

Even though my dad was feeling better, he still tired easily and gravitated toward his easy chair. So after breakfast and presents we gathered in the den and settled down for a Christmas movie marathon of whatever was showing on cable—*Elf, A Christmas Story*, and some iteration of *The Santa Clause*—interspersed with commercials for medications, hearing aids, and diabetes monitors. (This gave me time to answer all those "Sorry to bother you over the holidays" emails rolling in from subordinates and superiors alike.) It was actually quite cozy and I didn't want it to end, but to my disappointment Moose's flight was not canceled.

<Landed> came the dreaded text around 3 p.m.

I gave his text a thumbs up.

<Pick up kids on way home> He couldn't be bothered with complete sentences.

<No need. I'll bring them over around 5. I'd like to say hi to your folks.> *Also, if my mother sees you she might come at you, and she's been working out.* I didn't wait for his reply and put the phone in my purse. I would regret that before too long.

It was already almost dark on the half-hour drive over. The rental car smelled like fake leather and strawberry air freshener. The kids were quiet.

"Are you guys ok?"

"Yeah," Kelsey said, "just a little app... apprehensive? Like, when you're not sure how things will go?"

"Oh, good word! Yes, that seems natural. But I'm sure it's going to be great." I squeezed her knee. She didn't say anything more, so I turned my attention toward my firstborn. "Eliot?"

"What?" I could hear him frowning.

"Are you also apprehensive?"

"I'm fine."

"Well," I sighed, "not that you need my permission, but you guys should... I really hope you have a great time with your dad and Poppy and Nonna and your cousins and every-thing. They love you and you deserve to have fun, ok?"

"Ok."

"Whatever."

"Will you be ok with Gran and Gramps?" Kelsey asked.

"Of course! Don't worry about me. I have plenty of work to do and I'm going to see some old friends tomorrow, too." I tried to sound more cheerful than I felt.

There had been snow recently and the roads were patchy and winding so I stopped talking and focused on driving till we arrived at the vinyl-sided split-level that Moose had grown up in. We all got out and the kids pulled their bags out of the trunk. Still in the cold, I hugged them and told them I loved them, and then we walked to the front door.

When it opened, Moose's parents stood there together. *Does he think he needs a line of protection against me?* I tried to shake off my resentment. We squeezed into the front hall and said our hellos. I still had warm feelings about my ex-in-laws and was genuinely happy to be able to hug them again. They looked apologetic—or was it apprehensive—but no one said anything about the rupture in our familial ties. What was there to say?

"Dad!" Kelsey shouted after greeting her grandparents, who suddenly parted like the Red Sea. Moose stood behind them in the kitchen doorway and she ran into his arms. He swooped her up as if she were still a tiny child.

"Hey, little mouse!" He put her down. "Oh my god, you're so tall! And you—come here, my man." Eliot said nothing but I could almost see him melt into his father's hug. My chest ached for him.

The grandparents hung up coats and grabbed bags and bustled the kids off into the kitchen, leaving Moose and me alone in the front hall.

"Hey, Jen." He was smiling but his eyes were shifty. *Dude, I'm not gonna hit you.* He looked pretty much as he did last summer, but there was definitely something different about him. In place of my nerdy IT guy was a chilled-out man, tanned and wiry, with a stubbly salt-and-pepper beard, annoyingly fetching. He was wearing cargo pants and a linen shirt with a puffer vest...and a Santa hat. *Ok, maybe I will hit you.* My heart pounded in warning like a rabbit's foot.

"Hello, Moose."

"What happened to your face?" *Because of course he would.*

"Long story. How was your flight?"

"Fine, no problems. Except, um..."

"What?"

"Well, Amber was a little uncomfortable."

"Amber?" My face flushed. "Uncomfortable?" I immediately knew.

He took in a sharp breath and grimaced. He was spared having to explain when an athletic young woman came out of the powder room into the hallway, a KN95 mask on her face, a Santa hat on her head, and her belly protruding from her otherwise svelte body through a stretchy tunic.

He always wanted a third child.

"Oh! Hi." Her voice was muffled, her eyes more deer-in-headlights than smiling. I stared, my eyes hot and starting to water.

"Amber, this is Jen. Jen, Amber."

"I..." My bladder had already been complaining on the way over and now my bowels turned to jelly. I ran past Amber into the powder room she had just vacated and unbuttoned my jeans in a frenzy. The toilet seat was open and the water in it was still faintly rippling. The room smelled like shampoo, like her, like the other woman—young, nubile, desirable, a fertile field for my husband's seed. My guts rebelled against this reality. I tried desperately to catch my breath through my mouth, without smelling the mix of Amber and my own humiliation. I grabbed an obscenely large wad of toilet paper and bunched it up over my nose and mouth. Tears flowed down my face. *You asshole. You absolute fucking fuck of a fucking asshole. You couldn't have at least warned me?*

After a few minutes I cleaned myself up, splashed cold water on my face, and steeled myself to run the execrable distance from the powder room to the front door. There would be no polite farewells. I saw my saggy, bruised, scarred, blotchy face in the mirror, the coarse, crooked white hairs popping up from the top of my scalp. I cursed myself for making a scene like some ridiculous, middle-aged Karen. *Get it together, Jen, you can fall apart later.* When I finally exited the powder room Moose was standing alone in the front hall. I sped straight past him out the front door toward the car.

"Jen, come on," he pleaded, following me out into the cold night, "can't we talk about this?"

I spun around to face him. "Talk about this?" I shouted. "Now? She's like, at least five months pregnant! You could've fucking warned me!"

"I sent you a text!"

"A text?!"

"I'm sorry!" He whinged, probably more annoyed about getting caught than actually sorry. He reminded me of Eliot.

"No you're not!" I yelled. "If you were sorry you wouldn't have done any of this."

"Jen…"

"Grow up, Moose!"

I turned to make my escape and the next thing I knew I was slipping—again falling in slow motion. My right foot was in the air—*How does this keep happening?*—just before I landed hard on my tailbone. *That's gonna hurt tomorrow.* Then I was lying flat on my back in the driveway. The sky was perfectly clear. The stars were impossibly bright, the moon a half circle. *Waning gibbous. From the Latin for hump.*

My breath puffed out in front of my face, clouding the heavenly bodies once, twice.

"Oh my god, Jen, are you ok?" Time started up again as Moose's goddamn handsome tan stubbly face—the face of the man who used to love me and now loved some pregnant lady—blocked out the moon. *As if this could get any worse.* I wanted it to end immediately.

"Help me up."

I accepted his help to the car, my tailbone screaming. I gingerly sat down and slammed the door, almost catching him in it. I heard him saying something through the window but wouldn't look at him or listen.

Without another word, I started the car, put on my seatbelt, and backed out of the driveway as carefully as I could. I spent the drive back to my folks' crying, moaning in pain, and trying to sort out my spinning head. *How could you? How fucking could you?* When I got to my parents' I texted Jamie from the driveway.

<She's pregnant.> Was she still out for Chinese with her friends?

I wasn't ready to face my parents yet, so despite the throbbing pain in my hips and lower back, I took a slow walk around the neighborhood and tried to compose myself. The cold on my wrecked face was a welcome sensation. I walked in the middle of the street to avoid icy sidewalks, looking at the lights on all the houses. It was a little after 6:00 and families were still celebrating—some I had known all my life, and a few others I didn't know at all. I could see into their dining rooms or living rooms, warm and cozy and flickering with light and activity. Outside the Ricardis' house my phone buzzed.

<Oh, sweetie. [broken heart] I'm so sorry. Wanna talk?>

I started crying again, relieved and grateful that someone cared.

<Not yet, but thank you. [grateful hands] I'll tell you EVERYTHING when I get home.>

When I finally went inside, I could hear the sounds of my mom puttering in the kitchen and whatever sport my dad was watching, probably some golf tournament rerun. I ran straight upstairs and—after stopping in the bathroom— dropped myself on the bed. I couldn't bear to tell them about Amber, or even about the fact that I had fallen again. It would only make them worry.

I was just deciding I would take some pain medicine for now and wait till they went to bed so I could get a drink, when I heard a knock.

My dad peeked his head in. He always had a good sense of when it wasn't a job for Mom.

"Are you ok, Jenbug?"

"Yeah." I reminded myself of Eliot.

"Your mom made your favorite—spaghetti." That hadn't been my favorite since I was a kid, but whatever. It meant she understood that tonight was hard for me.

"I'll be ok, Dad. I just need a minute."

"Ok, sweetie." After a pause he added, "Do you need a hug?" *You do, in fact.*

"Yes, please." I groaned as I pushed myself off the bed, still wearing my coat. I limped over to my dad, who put his big, sweatered arms around me.

"How could he, Daddy?" I sobbed into his shoulder.

"I know, Jenbug, I know. I'm so sorry."

Early the next morning, after I had snored myself awake but was still in bed, Moose texted me.

<Jen can't we talk?>

When I opened up the thread, I saw that he had indeed tried to stop me from going to his parents' last night. <not a good idea> he had written, followed up by <Jen> and <Are you there>. I wanted badly to ignore him, but after telling him to grow up I felt obligated to send at least a brief reply.

<Good morning, Moose. I'm not ready to talk.> Then I added, <I'll be in touch later.> *How much later, Jen?* I had absolutely no idea.

<Ok sorry again>

Fuck you, Moose.

I was furious with him for turning me into some harpy. In my entire life, I had never been this full of rage. I hated myself for letting him get the better of me.

I worked most of the day, taking breaks to have coffee and lunch with my parents. I had plans for a Boxing Day mini-reunion with some of my old high school gang that evening.

Even though most of us had always lived within an hour or two of our hometown, work and parenthood and everyday life had curtailed our getting together except every five or ten years, usually at reunions. I had been lucky in my high school friends and still liked most of them (even after the revealing past few years, when all political tact had flown out the window), so even though my face was wrecked and my back was killing me, I was looking forward to seeing some people who were my friends before they were Moose's.

Everyone promised to take Covid home tests before meeting up in the afternoon at the Dark Horse Tavern—an overpriced, stuffy restaurant our parents used to frequent, with a slightly less stuffy bar where we could gather. As soon as I walked in I spotted a pair of fellow marching band nerds—our social drum majors who still lived locally and had arranged the whole thing—drinking wine on tall barstools. They stood up when they saw me coming.

"Ahh!" fake-screamed Brenda, an artist, stay-at-home-mom, and part-time yoga instructor. (Her husband, some kind of financier, wasn't in attendance.) She was even skinnier than she was in high school, skinny enough—I noted with envy—to wear tall suede boots over her jeans. I couldn't even get most boots to zip up over my naked calves.

"Oh my goooooood, Jeeeeeeen," fake-screamed Kimberly, an attorney, who was less skinny than Brenda but still skinnier than I, and looked wrinkle-free and beautifully polished in an oatmeal cashmere turtleneck and wool pleated slacks. *Stop it, Jen, no one cares. Anyway, someone has to look the worst. Think of it as performing a public service.*

"Smitty, dude, what happened to your face?" asked Thomas, who had entered not long after me, a marketer by day and a guitar player by night. *At least the stitches distract from how much weight you've gained.*

"Oh, you know, just a motorcycle accident."

He looked confused for a beat before pointing at me knowingly, his mouth wide open in a laugh. "Aaaahaaa-haaaaahaaaaaa!"

After a few more joyful meetings like these, I stopped worrying about my apple shape and frumpy outfit (a black button-down shirt and mom jeans, with a long charcoal cardigan I could add and subtract as my temperature fluctuated). Any anxiety I'd had about seeing them amid the current disaster that was my life was gone within a few minutes.

There was something about being with old friends—none of whom worked in higher ed—that put me at ease. No one expected me to act professional or sound smart. Somehow, knowing who I was in my teens meant they knew something like the real me, so faking anything wasn't necessary. We had all been young together, and were resilient enough to have survived this long. We still loved each other, and would always love each other, simply for that fact.

This included Michael, my old boyfriend. We'd been each other's "first" and had a hard break-up when we both left for college. He'd wanted to stay together long distance, but I wanted a fresh start. We hadn't talked at all in our twenties, but somewhere in our late 30s—right when Facebook was becoming a thing—we'd gotten back in touch now and then. After all these years what remained was fondness, and the comfort of knowing we'd already been through the worst.

"You look fantastic," I said after we hugged. Middle age really did look good on him.

"Thanks," he said. "You...look fantastic, too, except..." He pointed at his lip and we both laughed.

"Yeah, I had a little accident last week. Got my first stitches ever, whoo-hoo!" My hands made little rah-rah gestures.

"But you're ok?"

"Yeah, more or less."

"I heard about your break-up. I'm really sorry." He sounded genuine.

"Yeah, thanks. And last night I found out she's pregnant, so, yay!" He nodded sympathetically. "I feel so bad for my kids. It's not their fault their dad is having a midlife crisis. Or their mom, for that matter." A rueful laugh erupted unexpectedly from my throat. Alarm bells went off in my head as emotion welled up in my chest, so I shrugged it off and smiled. "Anyway, they're with him now at my in-laws'. Ex-in-laws. How about you? Didn't you retire?" He had made his millions selling insurance and retired at fifty.

"Yeah, but I still sit on a lot of corporate boards so I'm not totally settled down yet."

"I'm sure you're much in demand."

"More importantly, I'm gonna be a grandpa soon!" He had married and had kids right out of college. *The road not taken.*

"Seriously?"

"Yeah, Emma is six months pregnant." He looked genuinely pleased. "Wanna see some pictures?" We took out our phones and shared for a while, and it felt right.

I spent a couple of hours nursing a gin and tonic, making my rounds, and catching up on the biggest news in everyone's life. I relaxed and enjoyed myself. Their cultural references were my cultural references. They empathized about my divorce; some had been through it themselves. We commiserated about parenting teenagers while watching our parents deteriorate. We recalled our dorkiest memories and laughed at ourselves, then and now.

Driving home, I cried all the way again. *Good god, Jen, what's happening to you?* I had cried more in the last 24 hours than in the past four months.

I spent the last day of my trip in and out of zoom meetings with members of the college leadership, sometimes one-on-one, sometimes altogether. I dressed myself appropriately (even wore real pants, just in case I actually stood up on camera) and sat at my childhood desk, having rearranged the room toward the least unprofessional angle and removed a Duran Duran poster. A fan on the floor was set on low and pointed directly at my torso.

First, the student affairs committee needed to figure out what to do about yet another Covid semester, seeing as how we were about to bring a thousand young adults back from all around the state in the deep midwinter, into a county where case numbers were already in the red and our hospital was overwhelmed and understaffed. (The freaking *New York Times* had even cited it in an article about rural hospitals.)

Unsurprisingly, faculty, parents, and students had expressed mixed opinions about how to proceed. There was no way to make everyone happy, so I planned to ask for masks and boosters, per the latest public health guidelines, and leave it at that. No one was eager to be on the hook for making the call about boosters and masks, so I guessed as provost it was my job to at least have an informed opinion and go on record with it. I wanted to save what very little political capital I had for the budget meeting, and the longer-term issue of salary equity.

"Case numbers around here are still very high," I said when the time came, "and most of our students live on campus. Per my electronic survey of the faculty earlier this week, the vast majority still want everyone masked and vaccinated. MSU and Central Michigan are both requiring boosters for everyone on campus, so couldn't we do the same?"

"Yes, of course," Norm said, "it's extremely beneficial that we have already provided vaccine clinics for our community, and now boosters are widely available everywhere for anyone who wants one."

It took me a moment to translate what he'd said: No. One of Norm's favorite moves was to start by saying "yes" even if he immediately undercut it, as if he had taken some improv-for-administrators course.

"What I mean is," I tried again, "if we're going to require that everyone teach and work in person, it wouldn't be unreasonable or unprecedented for us to *require* that everyone get vaccinated and boosted, like our neighboring schools. Barring any Constitutionally-required exemption, of course." The president looked as if I hadn't said anything.

"We can't do that," responded the VP for Admissions, wearing an anxious smile. "It would kill us. We're a private school and we already have parents complaining about masks. A couple are threatening to pull their kids out, and we've already had a bunch of students withdraw after fall term." She studiously avoided the term "flunked out," which is what unprecedented numbers of college students were doing across the country.

"I understand that," I really did, and tried to keep my voice calm and kind, "but given the wide variety of responses from every direction, I think it's incumbent upon the college to make the smartest decision for the whole community, based on scientific recommendations." She shook her head but didn't reply. No one did. "If nothing else, we owe it to our employees to protect their health."

That was too much for the COO, who usually wore masks around his chin when he bothered to wear one at all. He was obviously exasperated by this ongoing conversation. "Look, Jennifer," (I felt myself flush and hadn't realized till just then how much I hated people who said "Look" before making a point) "our customers don't want to be forced to do anything, and for that matter neither do our employees. People who are still worried about it can wear masks, get vaccinated, and get boosters. Those who don't want to don't have to.

"And, Norm," he turned toward the president, "the college sure as heck can't keep paying for these things when people can get them elsewhere. If we require something, they'll expect us to provide it for free."

Norm cleared his throat. "This is a wonderful discussion, everyone," he said stiffly. "It's, ah, very important that we be able to, ah, share our ideas freely like this, and of course to, ah, get on the same page about what's best for the College of St. Margaret." He cleared his throat again. *Dude, get some Mucinex.* "I think at this point we'll stay the course, and we'll continue to post updated numbers at least once a week on the website."

As the VP of Student Affairs started talking about how we should all "remain vigilant about emotional wellness" on campus, I let myself fade into the background. I was disappointed but not a bit surprised. I would have to settle for providing continued flexibility in the sphere where I had any authority—letting instructors make decisions about their own classes, within reason, and being supportive of students who ran into trouble.

The next meeting was a budget update for just the president's cabinet—me and a whole bunch of other people with acronyms for job titles. It started with a shared-screen presentation by the CFO, a small, timid man who reminded me of a rabbit, to tell us there was good news. We were operating under budget, thanks to all the retirements, resignations, and cuts of the past year, and the fact that the endowment was still growing.

"So we've decided," Norm said when the CFO concluded, "that a portion of the surplus will be distributed as $500 bonuses to all employees." I looked at the COO in his tiny Brady Bunch square; based on his expression, this had not been his idea. "We hope that this will be a show of appreciation for the sacrifices everyone has made in the past couple of years."

I raised my hand and unmuted myself. "Norm, if I may?"

"Of course, Jennifer, go ahead."

"Thank you so much for the report and this is a really nice gesture. I think people will be grateful. I wonder if it might be possible for us to think longer-term about the budget, and particularly salary equity. I've noticed there are some real problems in the academic sector, especially among mid-career faculty, that need to be addressed pretty quickly."

Before Norm could answer the COO broke in.

"Look," *So help me god, dude, I'm gonna punch you in the throat,* "this is a one-time deal, and for the record I'm against it, as Norm already knows. We have no idea how long the surplus will last and now is not the time to be adding to our operating expenses. If anything, the surplus should be spent on marketing and recruiting."

"Yes, it is always wise to be cautious and conservative with expenditures," Norm said, "but in this extraordinary case I do think it's important to acknowledge the extraordinary efforts of our community to keep the college on track." The COO muted himself and backed down. *Wow, Norm, I didn't know you had it in you.*

"I whole-heartedly agree," I said. "I think it's a really good short-term plan, and I'd like us to talk next about long-term issues." The COO shook his head. Ignoring him, I said, "Norm, maybe you and I can talk about faculty salaries and come up with a proposal before the next cabinet meeting?"

"Yes, of course."

I muted myself and counted it a win.

By the time the VP for Advancement asked us all to donate to the College's spring fundraising campaign, I was drafting an email in my head to send to my sector about the coming semester. It would need to strike the proper tone, not throwing the president under the bus, but also letting people know I was willing to accommodate individual needs where possible. I could already predict the responses I would get. Maybe if I waited till after the president's announcement about bonuses things would go more smoothly.

It was going to be another long week.

Chapter 16

Screaming In the New Year

The time came to go "home" to Michigan. Leaving my parents was hard, especially my frail dad, and I cried again, all the way back to Newark airport in my strawberry-scented rental cry-mobile.

I saw Moose briefly when he dropped the kids off at the airport. Kelsey ran up and hugged me. Eliot stood near enough for me to put my arms around him briefly. I told them it was so good to see them and assured Moose I'd be in touch.

"Well, how was your visit?" I asked after we were through security.

"It was good," Kelsey said.

"I'm gonna go get a bagel," Eliot said. *That good, huh?*

"Do you have money?" I took his inaudible response for a yes. "See you at the gate." I turned my attention back to my daughter.

"What'd you do?"

"Um, I dunno, mostly hung out with Nonna and Poppy and played games and stuff." I could tell she was trying to avoid mentioning Moose.

"Was it good to see your dad?"

"Yeah." She sounded tentative. "He seems different. He was kind of, like, trying too hard, y'know? Like he wanted to act cool or something." That was unexpected.

"Huh," I said, "I guess this is all a little weird for him too."

"Yeah. And Amber's kinda weird."

"In what way?" *Besides being a home-wrecking little bitch?*

"She was kind of, like, whiney or something? Like, she kept making Dad do all these things for her, like wait on her and stuff."

"Well, she's pregnant. That can be hard on a body."

"Maybe. But she didn't seem like a mom at all. Not like you."

That's probably the point—someone who's not like me. "She'll be a mom soon enough. It changes everything."

"Mmm."

"Are you excited about the baby? You'll finally get to be a big sister."

"Yeah." She beamed so genuinely I could feel my heart cracking open.

Our flight was several hours delayed, so I fielded emails in the gate area, guarding my kids' stuff in between bathroom trips, while they alternately hunted for food and sat watching their phones. I laughed to myself, imagining an absurd sped-up video of the three of us with a Benny Hill soundtrack.

I hadn't slept well lately so I conked out on the flight in my middle seat, flanked by Kelsey at the window and Eliot on the aisle, grateful for the mask to cover my inevitable drooling. I strongly encouraged Eliot to drive us home from Detroit so he could get some highway driving experience near a big city. It probably wasn't great for our relationship, but we made it home alive and I hoped it had built his confidence behind the wheel a little.

I slept hard for a few hours and woke up around 4:00 a.m. It was new year's eve. I got up and went to the kitchen, made some coffee, and sat down with my laptop. I needed to catch up on new crises that had bubbled up overnight, along with some old, festering crises that wouldn't go away without the provost's intervention. The endless supply never ceased to amaze. Forget about trying to predict and ward off problems—I was drinking from a firehose.

Had I not been so busy I might have felt guilty about all the times I had criticized my past bosses.

I had promised Kelsey we would spend the day in our pajamas having an *Anne of Green Gables* marathon—the 1985 series, not that millennial nonsense-with-an-e. I stopped working when she got up around 9:00 so we could mix up a plum cake for breakfast. (I found a recipe online and figured the "dried plums" made it semi-healthy.) It was not the season for raspberry cordial so she would settle for raspberry tea.

When the cake went into the oven I texted Jamie. Having not been a teenage girl in the 80s, she had missed out and was excited to broaden her Gen X cultural references. Plus we'd missed her.

<We're almost ready for Anne. Come over whenever! Pajamas welcome.>

She responded with a gif of Moira Rose in a shiny gown, cat-walking through a flock of birds. My face smiled involuntarily and a warm bubble filled my chest. I suddenly couldn't wait even five more minutes to see her. Eliot interrupted my reverie.

"What the fuck happened to Betty White?" He stood in the kitchen doorway looking as if he was accusing me of something. "She was fine one day and now she's dead. Did she fall down the stairs or something?"

"I don't know," I said after processing his non sequitur. "She was 99 years old. People just have to die at some point." He looked genuinely disturbed. "If it makes you feel better, I read that she used to say, after people died, 'Now they know the secret.' So, now she knows the secret."

"So weird." He shook his head, ignoring my anecdote, and moved toward the pantry for some cereal. "What are you making?"

"Plum cake!" Kelsey answered with a little jig.

"Anyway," I asked, "why do you even know Betty White?"

"Everyone knows Betty White."

"Yeah, but I mean, what do you know her from?"

"Nothing, you just know about Betty White." He looked off into the distance for a few beats. "I guess *Community* might have been the first time I saw her in anything, but even then I already knew she was Betty White."

I found myself feeling jealous of this beautiful dead woman who had so captured my son's attention. She was never not gorgeous, never got fat, was always hilarious, and I'll bet she never had to answer emails about squalid living conditions for laboratory rats.

When Jamie arrived there were hugs all around. Under her coat she was radiant in ice blue silk pajamas with stylized zebras on them, supplemented by a fuzzy black vest and a simple, black cashmere beanie perched on her head. I devoured the sight of her.

We milled about in the kitchen for a while, drinking coffee and waiting for the cake. I let the kids fill her in on our holiday. Eliot didn't say much but he hung around. When Kelsey got to the part about Amber being pregnant, Jamie's eyebrows popped up and we briefly locked eyes.

Later, as we all moved into the living room, Jamie put her arm around my shoulders and whispered, "Oh my god, Jen." I looked at her and her eyes were full of tenderness. *I feel seen.*

"I know. I don't know why I was surprised. I should have known."

"When is she due?"

"I didn't ask," I said, "but I'm guessing it's not long from now, which means…" The lump in my throat stopped me from finishing.

"Oh sweetie," she said, drawing me into a full hug. I let myself lean into her till I was afraid I might lose it. I pulled away, rubbed my eyes, and sniffed.

"Shall we drown our sorrows in TV and cake?" she said.

"Yes, please."

Three of us assembled ourselves on the sofa and Eliot scurried upstairs. Getting to watch an old favorite show—

without guilt, because it counted as quality time—was one of the best things about having a teenage daughter.

Anne of Green Gables had always been a balm for my soul. Anne and Diana had comforted me almost like real friends during my moodiest high school years, and Gilbert Blythe was a dashing suitor. My only complaint back then was how long Anne punished Gilbert before admitting she was in love with him. I guess Kelsey was right—I had indeed been boy crazy. In fact I was boy crazy right up until the moment I decided to marry Moose, finally calming that restless part of me so I could focus on other things.

"I'm excited to see what all the fuss is about," Jamie said to Kelsey, as she arranged Mennonite doughnuts on a plate.

"Omigod, it's so good, you will LOVE it!" Kelsey said.

"What's it about?"

"It's about an orphan who goes to live with these old people."

I added, "And it's about bosom friends."

"I'm sorry, what?" Jamie did a double take. "Like 'Bosom Buddies'?"

I laughed.

"What's 'Bosom Buddies'?" asked my Gen Z daughter.

"It's the mildly inappropriate but strangely endearing show about men in drag that made Tom Hanks a star back in the 80s," Jamie answered.

"Oh." Kelsey took a bite of her cake.

"I promise it is nothing like 'Bosom Buddies,'" I said. "A bosom friend is like a best friend, a 'kindred spirit.' Someone you know you're going to love from the second you meet them. It's how Anne refers to her friend Diana."

"Oh!" Jamie's eyes sparkled, "That's how I felt when I met you!"

I felt a little flop in my chest and a stupid smile spread across my face. "Same!"

Midway through the series, Anne and Diana stood on a sand dune in the late afternoon light, looking out over the sea. Anne said, "This is the last of the Queen Anne's lace of the summer," and gently put a stalk in Diana's jet-black tresses.

With a sigh Kelsey said, "I miss the shore."

"Which shore?" Jamie asked. I loved that she always followed up, even on comments that were seemingly throwaways.

"The Jersey Shore," Kelsey replied. "I used to go there a lot during the summer with my friends, to Belmar and Ocean City and Island Beach State Park." She thought for a moment. "I loved the hugeness of the ocean. It really made me think about the meaning of life." I had never heard her say that before.

"Well you know," Jamie said, "you live near America's 'third coast' now. It's not saltwater, but maybe you could get your big water fix at Lake Michigan."

"Where's Lake Michigan?" Kelsey asked.

Jamie chuckled lightly before realizing it wasn't a joke. "It's...just a little west of here." She pointed toward the window.

"But is it really big, like that?" Kelsey pointed at the TV. "Like where you can't even see the other side?"

Jamie bolted upright, causing Fiona to leap from her lap. "Have you never seen a Great Lake?" Kelsey shook her head. Jamie looked at me as if I was guilty of the worst neglect.

"I really haven't either," I shrugged. "I mean, I've flown to Chicago for conferences so I know there's a lake there, but..."

"Seriously?"

"Well it was always winter," I protested, laughing. "It's not like I was hanging out on the beach!" I was reminded of that old cartoon of the 'New Yorker's view of the world' that basically skipped from the Hudson River to the Pacific Ocean, with a little patch of farmland in between. "And we moved here four months ago and I basically started working about two seconds later so we haven't done much exploring!"

"You literally! live! on a peninsula!" She clapped on literally, live, and peninsula, and then threw up her hands. "That's it. Road trip. Tomorrow. I'm driving. No excuses. The boy is coming too. This is happening." Jamie settled elegantly back into the sofa and rearranged her blanket. Kelsey and I looked at each other and laughed. It was a plan.

When *Anne* was over we made a big pot of spaghetti for dinner. Jamie had brought four party tiaras and we all put them on while the water boiled—even Eliot, who had drifted in and out of the living room all afternoon. She and I didn't want to stay up till midnight, so she popped open a bottle of alcohol-free champagne and filled four flutes she had brought with her. "Happy new year!" she shouted. Kelsey and I responded in kind. Eliot added a half-hearted, "Yaaaay."

"If we were at my house I would have thrown glitter," Jamie said, flinging imaginary handfuls as she spoke, "but I didn't want to make a mess at your house."

"You know glitter is like, really bad for the environment, right?" Eliot said.

"Don't make me regret inviting you down here, young man," She frowned exaggeratedly, shaking a fist in his direction. That got a half smile out of him. "And I'll have you know," she added, "I got some eco-friendly, biodegradable, plant-based glitter. So there."

New Year's Day was a Saturday, and it was freezing cold. Jamie and Deirdre picked us up—literally drove across the street into our driveway—with the Subaru already warmed up. There were travel mugs of hot coffee in the front center console and hot chocolate in the backseat cup holders. She had warned us all to put on lots of layers, and had neverthe-less come prepared with extra scarves, hats, and blankets to share. Dierdre sat happily in back between the kids, wear-ing an iridescent silver puffy jacket with a faux fur collar. While we were all getting settled, Jamie got the music and the map ready. She had downloaded the brand-new ABBA album to play on the car stereo.

"Have you heard this yet?" I had not. "It's of course not as good as their classic stuff but it's still a blast. Everybody buckled in?" The kids and I answered in the affirmative. "Saugatuck here we come!" she sang, backing carefully out of the driveway. "You are going to love it. It used to be an artists' colony, and it's still absolutely adorable even though it's super touristy now."

It was too cold for snow, as well as too cold for most mortals to travel anywhere, so the roads were almost empty. When we arrived, Saugatuck felt like a ghost town. Every-thing was closed because of the holiday, but Jamie had spent a lot of time there and wanted us to see it. After we layered on our winter gear and Deirdre went into a pouch on Jamie's front, we wandered down the middle of the streets, between piles of old snow and rows of colorful Victorians, brick storefronts, and wooden signs blowing sleepily over closed doorways. We window-shopped at tourist shops and art galleries, and stopped to read menus at restaurants. At one fancy-looking place called Bowdie's Jamie said, "I love this place! Oooh, bone marrow."

"People eat bone marrow?" Eliot asked, looking horrified.

"Of course! Waste not, want not, right? It's full of collagen so it's healthy for your joints and bones and skin. Spread on crusty French bread? Mmmm, it's marvelous." She closed her eyes thinking about it.

"Disgusting."

"Philistine."

I laughed, bouncing from foot to foot as this exchange took place, trying to stay warm, hyper-aware of Jamie's adorable smile lines. Deirdre's bug-eyes peeked miserably out of a gap in her pouch. She didn't love the cold as much as Jamie did.

After making a loop around the main downtown blocks and up the Kalamazoo river, we piled back into the car and headed over to the lake shore. We parked in a public lot and Jamie warned us all to bring blankets. The kids balked but she said, "Trust me on this one," so we obeyed and followed her.

Surrounded by mounds of sand and snow, sprinkled with hairy tufts of tall dead grasses, we could feel the wind from the lake before we could see it. With effort, we braced ourselves and climbed up a shifting hill between two peaks. Then there she was, Lake Michigan, in all her splendor.

The view took my breath away—and not just because the stabbing wind made me feel a whole new level of cold. The lake was indeed every bit as impressive as the ocean, endless and blue-gray, raging and noisy, whitecaps crashing one after another under a steely sky, no hint of land on the horizon. We walked close to where the water met the sand.

The fact that the beach was absolutely empty of human beings—something that almost never happened in New Jersey—gave the whole thing an added sense of beauty and awe. *Mysterium tremendum et fascinans*, I thought, weirdly reminded of a phrase I'd learned way back in a college religion class. I pulled my blanket tightly around me.

Suddenly Kelsey screamed, snapping me out of my trance. I turned frantically toward her, imagining a murderer approaching. Or a sea monster.

"What is it?" My voice wobbled with my chattering teeth. Her cheeks were tinged blue.

"I just felt like screaming." She laughed maniacally, the sound whipping away from us on the vicious, careless wind.

Jamie laughed too and said, "That's a great idea." Then she screamed, followed by a low belly laugh. Kelsey screamed again, and Jamie joined her, a soprano and tenor in harmony. I stood gaping stupidly at them.

"Come on, Mom, scream!"

"Do it, Jen, it feels great!"

I felt embarrassed, but looked around on the beach to confirm that there were no witnesses. I met Eliot's horrified eyes, pleading with me. *Sorry, kid,* I thought, before opening my mouth and letting a half-hearted holler emerge.

"Jesus," Eliot said, hightailing it away from us. I expected him to head back to the car, but he stopped and paced uncomfortably just short of the sand mounds, watching us but hiding from the imaginary judges who seemed to follow him everywhere.

"Come on, Jen, you can do better than that. Let it out!" Jamie and Kelsey screamed again.

I turned my back to my son and faced the water, trying again. It took me a minute to get going, but once I did,

I didn't want to stop. My jaw dropped lower, my throat opened wider, and relief swept through my whole body. I wanted Chicago to hear me.

The three of us kept hurling our stress and anxiety and sadness and joy at the lake for a while longer, our voices disappearing into the forgiving crashing of the waves. The wind poked holes in our faces with mist and grains of sand, as our hair and blankets flapped out behind us. Deirdre blinked and shivered in long-suffering silence.

"Oh, I almost forgot!" Jamie took off a glove and reached into her buried pocket, pulling out a bag of what I assumed was eco-friendly glitter. "Want some?"

I declined, too cold to move my hands, but Kelsey removed her mitten to receive a handful. As Jamie tried to pour some into her open hand, most of it was whipped away instantly, eliciting more screams and laughter. She ended up just shaking the bag out around us. Most of it vanished into the air and sand and snow, never to be seen again. Some of it landed on the two beloved faces before me, adding sparkle to already overwhelming beauty. I almost couldn't stand it.

"Ohhhhhh myyyyyy gooooooood," my scream morphed into an exclamation, "it's freezing out here, let's go!" We ran awkwardly in the sand back toward Eliot, who waited for us to pass, and then over the dunes toward the car, laughing all the way. The doors were still locked so we couldn't get in, which made us laugh even more while Jamie struggled to find her keys.

"Get in, get in," she said as the locks clicked open. She started the car, turned the heater on high, unharnessed Deirdre and sent her into the welcoming arms of the back seat. Then she got back out of the car, went to the rear and opened it, retrieved a picnic basket, and came back into the front seat with a "Whew." The basket rested on the center console.

"Lunchtime!" she sang. Inside were sandwiches wrapped in beeswax cloths (I hoped Eliot would approve) and appealingly bright orange clementines, which she distributed all around. There was another a big thermos of hot chocolate, which I poured into the kids' travel cups one at a time, then ours. I'd left a little coffee in my cup that morning so the cocoa tasted like mocha.

"What...is that?" Eliot asked.

"It's vegan cheese, hummus, and sprouts." I loved that she had made a special sandwich for my boy.

"No, that," he said, nodding at Kelsey's sandwich.

"It looks like salami on cinnamon raisin bread," Kelsey said, sounding puzzled.

"Yes! With salted European butter!" Jamie added.

"Seriously?" Eliot followed up.

"Seriously," Jamie said. "It's delicious. I once had it at a street fair in Hamburg and I've never forgotten it. It's now my favorite cold-weather picnic food." I couldn't help smiling at the idea of having a favorite as specific as cold-weather picnic food.

"What's your favorite hot-weather picnic food?" I asked. "Or your favorite cold-weather restaurant food?"

Jamie munched thoughtfully. "My favorite hot-weather picnic food is definitely cucumber and dill sandwiches. Ooo, and watermelon." She thought some more. "I'll say my favorite cold-weather restaurant food is bone marrow, but that's probably because we just saw it on the menu. Oh by the way, here's a bag for the clementine peels." She handed a green compost bag to me and I passed it to the back seat.

After chewing on a bite of her sandwich, Kelsey said, "It's pretty good." Then she asked, "What does Deirdre get for lunch?"

"A sandwich, of course! She loves these. It reminds her of her past lives in Germany."

"She lived in Germany before?" Kelsey asked.

"Oh at least once," Jamie said with conviction. "Maybe a few times, before we knew each other. It's hard to know because she's not talking."

Kelsey looked worried until she decided Jamie was joking. She let out a light-hearted giggle that I hadn't heard in a while. Then, leaning back against her seat with a big sigh, she said, "That. Was awesome."

"It really was." I turned to Jamie and said earnestly, "Thank you for bringing us."

"Yeah, thanks," Kelsey added.

"You're most welcome, my dears. Now you're no longer Great Lakes virgins." That got a "Hehe" out of Eliot and an "Ew" out of Kelsey.

On the drive home, Kelsey prevailed upon Jamie to play her Harry Styles playlist instead of ABBA. Both kids and the dog eventually fell asleep in the back, Deirdre with her head on Eliot's thigh, Kelsey with her head on Deirdre. I looked stealthily at Eliot, sleeping with his head against the window, while I could. Surrendered to sleep, he resembled the sweet, trusting little boy he used to be. *Maybe... we can... find a... place to feel good*, Harry sang, *and we can treat people with kindness... find a place to feel good.*

While they slept, I filled Jamie in on the basic outlines of the holiday family drama, keeping my voice and my emotions down. I tried to make the whole thing sound funny so she wouldn't know how utterly pathetic I really felt.

"When do you think you'll talk to him?" Jamie asked.

"I don't know. I still..." My voice broke. *I still don't think I can talk to him without losing it.*

"You'll talk to him when you're ready."

"Yeah." *I can't imagine ever being ready.*

Later in January I found myself sitting on Eliot's bed with my laptop while he sat at his computer, staring at the screen. I was trying hard to take deep breaths and watch the snow flurries and not create more stressful vibes in the room than were already floating around. He was finishing his Common Application. I had emailed him all the essay and short-answer prompts from the website, and he was supposedly working on his answers, which he could email back to me for proofreading and plugging into the forms.

"How about I hire a college counselor to help you with all this?" I had asked him back in August. I desperately didn't want to be a helicopter parent, or a snowplow parent, or whatever metaphor for failure the moms of my generation were currently being.

"No way."

"It's either that or you'll have me nagging you to get stuff done."

"Fine."

"Really? You're choosing to have me nag you?"

"I don't want some stranger nagging me."

So here we were, at the very last minute (he had already missed the early action deadlines), doing a thing I swore I would never do. *How did it come to this?* I had written my college application essay in the summer before my senior year of high school, and obsessively studied for the SAT. And now I had a kid who couldn't make himself do anything that might improve his chances of getting into the school of his choice, despite assuring me he did want to go to college —probably because he didn't know what else to do. It's not that I wanted him to go to a big name school, but even the least competitive colleges required a damn application.

I had urged him to apply to at least two of the state universities (Michigan seemed to have dozens of them, most of them struggling to find enough students), as well as a few colleges in the upper Midwest and the Northeast that were part of the same tuition-exchange group as St. Margaret's. Finally, after a long career of earning relatively crappy wages, my job was going to pay off in the form of cheaper school and lower debt for my kid.

"Come on, hon, it's getting late." I finally cracked after answering all my time-sensitive emails and watching him dick around for an hour. "Just start writing something. You can go back and fix it later."

"Oh really," he said, "is that how writing works?" Sometimes I wanted to punch him right in his stupid, sarcastic nose. I took a breath.

"I'm not the enemy here. I'm just trying to help."

"Well you're not helpful." He turned back to his computer. "I don't see why I can't just go to St. Margaret's." His voice was so low I almost missed it.

"Wait, what?" He didn't answer. I took a moment to process. "You want to go to St. Margaret's?"

"I don't know," he shrugged, still not looking at me, "why not?" My mouth dropped open in disbelief.

"I just assumed you would want to get as far away from home as possible."

"Whatever, it's fine."

The poor kid must have spent the last couple of years feeling like the ground underneath him was shifting like sand—pandemic, moving, divorce. Staying close to home (and to Anna, of course) probably sounded good after all the unwelcome changes that had befallen him in his short life. I wanted to kick myself for not having thought of it. *If it had been your idea he would have rejected it outright.*

"Well, ok then. That's actually great!" He finally looked at me. "You can go tuition-free and save a lot of money." He shrugged. "And they have rolling admissions so we—you can put this off till later."

"Ok," he said. His face had relaxed into a slightly less angry expression. I was liking the idea more and more.

"Kelsey will be thrilled! Plus," I added enthusiastically, "they have a cross country team that would probably be glad to have you."

"Hmm." I gave him a big dorky smile and he grimaced in return. I closed my laptop, bounced over to him, grabbed him around the shoulders and kissed him on top of the head. He didn't reciprocate my affection but he didn't pull away either.

"Awesome," I said, "I get to keep you around a while longer!" I was a little surprised at how relieved I felt. I had resigned myself to losing him, on top of everything else I had lost or was in the process of losing. I was elated that that might be put off for a few years.

"Mmmm kay," he said, patting my hand. "That will be enough for now."

I dutifully got out of his hair before he went back to being mad at me.

Chapter 17

Zoom, Zoom, Zooma Zoom

The first post-new-year's weekend in January was always the annual meeting of the Modern Language Association, which an article in the *Washington Post* called "the most important, and most heavily trafficked, gathering for scholars of literature and culture." It also said, "To make a career out of the humanities is to accept emergency as the norm" and to be "inevitably at home with ongoing crisis." *Tell us something we don't know.*

MLA had been an annual holiday in my professional and personal life since graduate school, except one year when I was very pregnant. It was the great scholarly get-together where I had given my first ever professional paper back in the 1990s ("The Veil upon Her Heart: Constance, Queen of Sicily in *Paradiso*"), where I had interviewed for faculty jobs (including Madison College), and where I had met with the editor of the academic press that had published my first and only book (*Dante's Women*, which cost $90 and had sold approximately 250 copies in 20 years). I had always shared a hotel room at MLA meetings with three of my grad school besties, a tradition we'd started when we were poor students. We still slept two to a bed and stocked our room with the cheapest possible red wine from the nearest convenience store, despite having grown up and gotten "real" jobs back in the early aughts—before higher ed had begun its death spiral in earnest, with language programs being ruthlessly culled, year after year.

In 2021 the annual meeting had been canceled due to Covid, and this year I couldn't justify going because of the demands of my new administrator role, not to mention single parenting. So apparently 2020 had been my last MLA. I wished I had known at the time. I would have savored it more—the miles of tables laden with obscure books, the chance meetings with old acquaintances and famous scholars, the panels on "Contemporary Perspectives and Adaptations of Dante's *Comedy*" or "Space and Mobility in Medieval and Renaissance Italian Literature, 1600-1900."

Anyway, that Friday I had a Zoom date with my roomies, all of whom were still faculty and lived within a reasonable train ride from Washington, DC.

"Hey, friends!" I sang, trying to sound cheerful as their images appeared on my screen. They shouted back in a disorderly chorus.

"How's it going?" I asked.

"Oh," said Melissa, waving her hand dismissively, "it's totally dead here." She was a professor of Russian languages and cultures at Boston University. She was kind of a big deal —one of the only people I knew who had actually moved up from one tenure-track job to an even better one. Her second book, a groundbreaking meta-study on the study of

Russian women's literature in American higher education, had won all kinds of scholarly awards. I was pretty sure she would chair the MLA executive council someday, especially now that Russia was back to being a main U.S. adversary (or hero, depending on your politics). She was tremendously driven, much more than the rest of us, and thrived on constant stress—at least until she got breast cancer a couple of years before. She tried to slow down after that but it just wasn't in her nature. "I guess most lit professors don't want to risk death for a dying profession. Go figure."

"Yeah, you're not missing anything," said Yasmine; "everyone's just watching the panels from their hotel rooms." She was the sole French professor at a no-name regional college in central Pennsylvania, where she also had to teach Arabic because she happened to speak it and there weren't enough students to support a full-time French professor anymore. "I gave a paper to three people! THREE! Hashtag winning!" She held up a glass of wine and took a drink. The two of them were sitting together on a bed. The frame bobbed around dizzily.

"It's so empty, even the book exhibit." Lesley's face was alone in a separate box on the screen. She was sitting on the other bed with her computer muted, so her voice was distant and seemed to come from Yasmine and Melissa's screen. "We miss you so much!"

"I miss you too," I said, suddenly feeling a lump in my throat. I willed it away. "Are you presenting, Les?"

"No," she said, "I'm supposed to be interviewing candidates for a one-year German position." She, a scholar of Spanish and Mexican culture in Philadelphia, was the lone tenured language professor left at her tiny women's college named after an obscure saint. She had watched her department gutted, losing job after job as her senior colleagues retired. The other languages—French and German—were temporary, year-to-year jobs. Hers would probably go that way too whenever she retired. Students, the "customers" of higher education—as the COO loved to remind me—just didn't care about studying languages anymore. "But I'm mostly doing that virtually, too, since almost no one is actually here in person."

"Oh, get this you guys," Yasmine interrupted, holding her phone up in front of her screen. "My dean just sent us a twenty-four page memo about stuff we have to put in our syllabi this semester. Our semester ALREADY STARTED!"

"What the fuck?" said Melissa.

"That's some bullshit," Lesley confirmed.

"She is just..." Yasmine read, "Listen, 'It is imperative for our retention efforts that we plan ahead'—PLAN AHEAD!—'and make use of the most IMPACTFUL practices.'" Everyone booed and laughed on cue. We all hated the rise of business-ese words like "impactful," even if they were technically OED-approved.

Lesley said in a child's voice, "Every time someone says 'impactful' a deano gets her wings."

"Hear, hear!" Melissa said. "Drink!" Everyone laughed and drank, including me. And then, before I knew what was happening, my laughs suddenly turned into tears.

"Oh no, what's wrong, baby girl?" Melissa asked.

"I'm sorry for making fun of deanos!" Lesley said, leaning into the camera. "I didn't mean you!"

Yasmine chimed in, "You are *nothing* like my dean, I'm sure of it!"

"It's not that," I said, "I just cry all the time now, apparently."

"You do? Why?"

Where to begin? "I hate missing time with you guys!"

"Awww, sweetie, we miss you too," Melissa said. "But seriously, what's wrong? Why are you crying all the time? Is it just 'cause of Moose?"

I gave into my self-pity. "It's everything! I'm old and fat and gross, and my husband left me, and my kids hate me and my faculty hate me and my boss hates me." I paused and sniffled as they cooed sympathetically. "And I only have one friend here and she's too cool for me and will probably dump me soon too."

"Babe," Melissa said, "you've been through a lot. But by the way, stop equating fat with gross. It's so Boomerish."

"I know."

"And white."

"I know." (This was not the first time we'd had such an exchange.)

"Tell us about your friend," Lesley interrupted diplomatically.

"Jamie," I said. "She's amazing. She owns a bookstore and she's funny and fun and my kids love her and for some reason seems to like hanging out with us." I told them about screaming into the stormy winds of Lake Michigan.

"She sounds like something good in your life," Lesley said.

"She is." *And, sidebar, I kind of have a crush on her.*

"So spend more time with her when you can."

"Yeah."

"And get a good therapist," said Yasmine.

"You'll get cancer if you don't take care of yourself, Jen," Melissa said. "Take it from me."

"I know."

"You probably also need to get laid, or at least get a good vibrator," added Lesley.

"Shut up!" We all laughed. "I just need to stop being an idiot."

"You're not an idiot," Melissa said. "You're just having a shitty year. Remember how bonkers I was during my cancer year? You've been through huge changes so it's no wonder you're feeling off!"

"And seriously, you're not gross so please stop saying that!" Lesley shouted. "Just because Moose is a dick doesn't mean there's something wrong with you."

"I know, I'm sorry. It's probably just lack of sleep."

"Oh my GOD, insomnia, don't even get me started!" said Yasmine. "Perimenopause is the absolute worst!"

I was eager to remove myself from the center of conversation. "What's going on?"

"Ugh," she scoffed, "what ISN'T going on? I can't sleep anymore, and I mean look at my face!" She leaned into the camera. "I have acne again! Like I'm 15!"

"Me too on insomnia," Melissa chimed in, "plus I have to pee constantly and I've lost all interest in sex. Ugh, and the brain fog...I thought for sure it was either chemo brain or long Covid but my doctor said it could also be menopause."

"Get hormone replacement, ladies, you'll never regret it," Lesley said. "My moods have totally regulated and I sleep like a baby. It's awesome."

"Really?" Yasmine asked. "I thought hormone replacement therapy caused cancer or blood clots or something."

"That's a myth perpetuated by the patriarchy," Lesley declared, as passionate as a college student who had just discovered feminism. "Men just don't want us to be happy if we're not procreating for them."

"I'm already taking too many anti-cancer hormone drugs," Melissa said. "Hey did I mention I finally found a Black doctor?" Melissa's dad was Russian but her mom was Black. "You cannot believe how much better it is! Like, she *actually believes me* when I tell her things about my body!"

"That's awesome!" I said. "Did your other doctors not believe you?"

"Never! White doctors see a Black woman and either don't care or don't believe she might actually be in pain. It's a widespread problem—there's all kinds of research on it. At least when I had cancer they believed I had an actual problem that had to be treated, but pain? Or hot flashes? Pssshh. They're like, 'Get over it.'"

"That's horrible," I said. "I had no idea."

"Yup. But my new doctor believes me and is willing to try some things. So I just started taking an SSRI that might help with the hot flashes."

"I hope it works," Lesley said.

Yasmine broke in, "Maybe perimenopause is my dean's problem. She and I should start a support group." More laughter and drinking.

Amid this "organ recital" (what my mom called it when old people sat around talking about their health ailments) it occurred to me that I couldn't actually remember having a period in Michigan. As I listened to them talking about their symptoms, I wondered if maybe my recent crying fits were at least partly hormonal, and not exclusively related to grief or the shit-show that was my current life.

After an hour and a half it was time to sign off. "I love you guys so much!" I said. "Thanks for calling."

"We love you!" they shouted. Melissa leaned in, kissed at the camera and said, "Seriously, find a therapist and a doctor. And maybe even some drugs – why not? You'll feel better."

"Yeah," said Yasmine, "you're not going to single-handedly solve the problem of big pharma by letting yourself be miserable."

I sat for a few minutes after they were gone, letting their beloved voices ring in my ears till they faded out. I was a little dizzy from the wine and the Zoom, and I had a headache from crying. I turned out the lights and fell asleep almost immediately.

I woke up a couple of hours later—a hot flash rather than a snore—and got up to go to the bathroom. There was light coming from under Eliot's door. I resisted the urge to tell him to go to bed. I peed, brushed my teeth, and went back to bed, lying in the dark thinking. It had indeed been shitty year, and I hadn't been taking care of myself. Apart from getting vaccines (and tooth repair, and stitches) I hadn't seen a medical professional since before the pandemic. I was well overdue for a mammogram and a pelvic exam, and wasn't I supposed to get a colonoscopy when I turned fifty?

What if it was possible to feel a little bit better than I had been feeling? I made a mental note to schedule some self-maintenance appointments in the very near future.

Chapter 18

The Menopausal Middle

When I opened my email on the Sunday before the semester started, I was reminded of Harry Potter's invitations to Hogwarts flying out of the fireplace at the Dursleys' house. There were dozens. Some of them I could quickly delete—meeting reminders, campus events, and the like— but others needed more attention.

The psychology department chair wanted to know when there would be a decision regarding a search for a replacement hire this year; I replied it was on my agenda to discuss with the president at our next one-on-one, along with all the other searches that I had determined we badly needed. The chair of the music department wanted to know if their adjunct instructors were eligible for professional development grants; I checked the manual and couldn't find any information either confirming or denying it, so I promised to put it on the agenda for the Tenure and Promotion Committee.

Most of the emails were things like this—faculty wanting to do their jobs well, but not having the information or the authority to make certain things happen that *had* to happen before they could complete their tasks. They needed me to do my job first. One email, though, made me gasp audibly.

"What?" Kelsey asked, startled. I didn't answer immediately, trying to process what I was reading. "Mom, what?" she repeated.

"One of the professors has ovarian cancer," I said. The email was from a nursing professor, who was probably in her late 50s. She wrote that she had been diagnosed with ovarian cancer, that she needed to undergo chemotherapy right away and surgery in a couple of months, and that she had already been in touch with HR about a medical leave. (Our HR officer was cc'd on the email.)

"Is that bad?" Kelsey asked.

"Very bad," I said. "It's almost always fatal, because it's almost never caught until it's too late."

"Oh," she replied solemnly.

"At least I think that's still true," I added, trying to remember if I'd heard anything about it recently. "The symptoms of ovarian cancer are basically the same as symptoms of other stuff. And no one has ever bothered to figure out an easy test for it, and insurance companies don't want to pay for expensive tests even if they actually work, so people basically just don't know they have it till they're already dying." Kelsey looked terrified.

I felt rage at the system welling up inside me and tried to shut it down so I could focus on how best to answer. An email for news this grave didn't seem like enough, but a sudden phone call from me might be unwelcome. I decided on a brief, empathetic reply right then, with the promise (and fair warning) of a follow-up phone call.

First thing Monday morning I called HR to make sure I knew what my responsibilities were. Then I called and talked to the nursing professor, who was understandably weepy, and weirdly apologetic about leaving the college in the lurch. I silently cursed capitalism for messing with humanity's priorities, and outwardly sought to reassure her that she was absolutely right to make beating cancer her number one project. I told her it was my job to handle the fallout at work, though I would always be grateful for any advice she had to offer. She did in fact have some leads on replacement teachers, which I gratefully accepted since I hadn't yet made any relevant contacts in the area.

My next call was to make a doctor's appointment. I hated going to doctors, but the Zoom call with my friends already had me thinking about how much I'd neglected my health, and news of an ovarian cancer diagnosis scared me enough to finally take action. I didn't want to wait for another emergency before forming a relationship with a medical professional. The non-dental equivalent of a broken tooth could potentially prove a lot more traumatic, and I didn't want the kids to have to suffer another major upheaval in their lives.

There was only one OB-GYN in town, the one where Anna's mother worked, so I decided to start with a general practitioner. Google sent me to Lake Family Practice, where all three of us could go, and which was in the college's health insurance network. There was only one doctor there, a DO—doctor of osteopathic medicine—rather than an MD. I had never heard of this before, but an internet search assured me that DOs were in fact "real" doctors, though comparatively more likely to end up doing primary care than specializing. I figured maybe it was a Midwestern thing. The doctor was a man and I really didn't want to get naked in front of male doctors anymore, so I requested an appointment with a female PA or NP. The earliest appointment was weeks away, February 28. *Why does that date sound familiar?* I couldn't remember so I booked it.

Weeks of snow and grey and emails and meetings seemed to fly by and soon it was late February. The appointment was first thing in the morning, so I took my kids to school and drove from there. Between the school and the doctor's office I got stuck waiting at a railroad crossing. I put the minivan in park so I could space out while waiting for the long freight train to pass—a giant-sized version of Eliot's old Thomas the Tank Engine sets. The radio droned on about Supreme Court justice replacements. A string of giant black cylinders marked NON-ODORIZED LIQUIFIED PETROLEUM GAS slowly dragged across the road. One battered white rectangle had been marked by an artist named "Atomik" in yellow, green, and orange graffiti, reminiscent of several African flags. I wondered where this train had come from, where it was going.

Next to me waited a large pick-up truck with a flat-bed trailer full of carousel horses on poles. I had a sudden memory of what it felt like to sit on a horse like that and bob up and down—how many years had it been since I rode one with my kids? At least a decade, probably. Had I already had my last carousel ride ever, and not even noticed? I sighed. Maybe I'd live long enough to have a grandkid.

Lake Family Practice looked like a brand-new building. After checking in I sat down facing a big fish tank, to fill out what felt like hundreds of questions on an iPad, about me and my family health history. When I was finished I checked out the multi-colored fish, swimming casually around their furniture. Above the tank was a television set playing a loop of silent ads with smiling faces and tips for good health. *Yes, in fact I did know that I'm at risk for Type 2 Diabetes, you smug SOB.*

Eventually I heard my name called by a young white woman in purple-patterned scrubs, who led me into the generic rabbit's warren of offices behind the reception area. She said hello but didn't smile and made virtually no eye contact. She measured my height (I wasn't shrinking yet), weight (*sweet Jesus*), and blood pressure (I had never understood how blood pressure numbers worked but even I knew those were higher than they should be). She then took me to an examination room where I had the choice of two chairs, one of them extra wide. I felt compelled to prove that I could still easily fit between the arms of the smaller one.

She asked me a few more questions before leaving with a promise of "Dr. Terri's" imminent arrival. Dr. Terri, a Nurse Practitioner, did indeed arrive promptly. She was a tall, athletic-looking white woman who might have been in her 30s or 40s (the Covid mask made such things hard to pinpoint), with a haircut reminiscent of Bat Benetar. *The 80s called*, I thought cattily, *they want their haircut back.*

"Good morning," she said, looking down at me and shaking my hand firmly in her thin, bony one. I tried to exchange pleasantries and weather reports with her while she washed her hands, but she was all business. When she settled down at the tiny desk with her laptop, her posture rigidly straight, she proceeded to go through a checklist, asking me a number of the same questions I had already answered, as well as a few new ones.

"Your blood pressure is a little high." She frowned at the laptop. "Is that typical for you?"

"I don't think so?" I felt suddenly like a child. "I'm not sure."

"We'll have to check when we get the records from your old doctor." She looked me in the eyes. "If this is typical we'll need to get it under control. Heart disease is the leading cause of death for women in the U.S., and hypertension puts you at risk."

"Ok." I sat up straighter to try to reclaim some dignity. "What causes it?"

"Any number of things," she said, "genetics mostly, but also stress, diet, age, weight gain..." She paused and then asked, "Is this a typical weight for you?"

"No! I've been the same weight for years. This," I gestured toward my torso, "has all happened in the last year or so."

"You'll want to keep that under control." *Ya think?* "Have you been unusually stressed?" I almost belly-laughed.

"Besides being a parent and a teacher in a pandemic?" She didn't even crack a smile so I reined myself in. "Well, also, my husband left me, I moved here, I started a new job, my dad's health is failing, and," I held up the five fingers upon which I had been counting, "I'm now parenting two teenagers all by myself, one of whom hates my guts. Does any of that count as unusual stress?"

"I see." She moved on. "Do you do regular breast exams on yourself?"

"No. I stopped after I read a study that they didn't result in any better outcomes than regular mammograms." That wasn't entirely true. I had *never* done regular breast exams, but I stopped *feeling guilty* about it after I read they didn't lead to better outcomes.

"So have you had a baseline mammogram?"

"Not yet," I admitted. "I was going to when I turned 50 in 2020 but then, you know." I shrugged. "That's partly why I'm here."

"When was your last pap smear?"

"Late 2019, I think."

"Do you still menstruate?"

"Yes?"

She raised an eyebrow and peered at my graying hair. "What was the date of your last period?"

"Well, it's been a while…" I scolded myself for not figuring this out before coming. I thought for a minute and then remembered.

Moose and I had scheduled a date night on our last wedding anniversary—our first night out alone together in more than a year. Three of us were vaccinated (Kelsey still wasn't eligible at that point, but she'd been going to school with the unvaxxed masses for months) so we figured we could risk a dinner out. I had scrubbed and shaved and trimmed myself all over so we could have sex afterwards—I couldn't remember the last time we'd done that either—and I'd put on an actual dress, a flattering red wrap with a low neckline that accentuated my new larger breasts while minimizing my new larger midriff.

Since it was a special occasion, we had gone a little farther afield to our favorite Italian place, the one that reminded me of the Grand Ticino in *Moonstruck*, and between dinner and dessert I had gone to the ladies' room and found blood in my panties. It wasn't a lot—lately I'd been having the kind of brown, clumpy, salty-smelling period I used to get in middle school when it was first getting started—but it was enough to put the kibosh on romance.

Moose had never been one for period sex. When I told him he'd seemed neither surprised nor disappointed. That made more sense now.

"Last May," I answered.

"Are you sexually active?"

"Not lately," I said.

"What do you mean lately? Months? Years?" I felt accused of something.

"Months."

Having completed her checklist she asked, "Are there any particular concerns you'd like to discuss today?"

We talked about ovarian cancer, colonoscopies, joint aches, blood panels, and my new fear that I probably had a brain tumor that was messing with my emotional equilibrium and my ability to remember things.

"Do you have frequent headaches?" she inquired. "Unexplained nausea or vomiting? Problems with vision? Loss of sensation in your limbs?" No, no, and no.

"But I can't sleep at night and I'm drowsy all day. I have brain fog and I'm really forgetful now, and I never was before. And lately I have terrible mood swings. I've been losing my temper a lot and even lashing out at people, and I've never been a person who does that."

"You're over 50. All of those symptoms are consistent with perimenopause," she shrugged without empathy. Ugh. It was exactly as my friends had suggested. "That's likely also what explains your excessive weight gain." *Suck it, skinny bitch.*

"Well is there anything I can do about it? Like maybe hormone replacement therapy?"

She stiffened. "Menopause is a perfectly natural stage of life and I can't recommend hormone replacement. If you want that I can refer you somewhere else."

I felt like a dog who'd been slapped. "Oh."

"You just need to exercise, drink more water, go to bed early, and avoid alcohol, fat, caffeine, and sugar. That will help with both the weight and the sleep issues. Given your weight you may also have sleep apnea, so you may need a CPAP." She was on a roll so I did not interrupt. "But if your blood pressure keeps going up you'll need medication for that. And if you're depressed, we can talk about SSRIs."

I thought it was weird that medications for all these other things were apparently fine, but hormone replacements were not. "All right." My face grew hot and I was having trouble looking her in the eye. "I just thought I should ask."

She then had me sit on the examination table where she looked in my eyes, ears, and throat, and listened to my heart and lungs. She had me lie down and unzip my pants. She pressed around my abdomen and asked if anything hurt. Then, apparently satisfied, she washed her hands again, packed up her laptop, and said the nurse would be back with all the paperwork for all my follow-up tests. I was still fully clothed.

"Do I need to change into something?" I asked.

"No," she said, "with women your age who aren't sexually active we no longer do a pelvic every year unless you have a specific complaint or a history of abnormal pap smears." I felt both relieved (absolutely no one enjoys the speculum) and insulted. *I must really be at the end of my useful life if even a pap smear is more than I deserve.*

I went through the motions of thanking her, thanking the assistant who came back with my flu shot and my paperwork, and thanking the woman at the counter who took my co-pay as I exited. Then, in what was apparently my new normal, I got into my car and burst into tears.

After getting myself together, I went into work. I checked in briefly with Fran to make sure there were no fires to put out, and then went into my office and closed the door. I didn't feel up to dealing with unnecessary interruptions.

I also had to recuperate before my next undesirable appointment of the day—with a divorce lawyer. I had learned that we couldn't legally start proceedings in Michigan till I had lived here for 180 days, so Monday, February 28 was the earliest possible day. I went to the bathroom and checked out my face and hair before logging on with a local family attorney named Monica (Jamie had known her since middle school and said she was a good person) to officially file what was called a "complaint for divorce."

"Hi, Jennifer." She had dyed red hair, cut short, and looked very put together.

"Hi, Monica." I did my best to smile. "Today's the day."

"Yes, it is. How are you feeling about it?" *Please don't ask me that.*

"I'm just ready to get it done."

"All right, well it's pretty straightforward." She walked me through the paperwork and next steps. "Because of your minor children, it's another six months before there can be a judgment. In the meantime, you and Matthew can work with a mediator to figure out any details. Is he likely to cause any problems regarding your shared assets?"

I thought for a minute.

"I don't think so. He's pretty ashamed of himself."

"Even so, sometimes people can be surprisingly difficult when they're feeling defensive. Because he has been the primary breadwinner during your marriage, you'll want to make sure to get your fair share. You have to think of yourself and your children, especially if his new partner is expecting." I resented these comments but reminded myself that it was her job to expect the worst and protect me—and especially my kids—from it. Still, it made me feel dirty to think about fighting over money with the person I made humans with and once vowed to love till I died.

"I think it will be fine," I said as confidently as I could. "I am also a breadwinner, even if I earn less than he does. I know he loves our kids and I'm really not interested in punishing him. I just need to move on."

"All right then, that should make things easier." She gave me some assignments and we finished our conversation. After hanging up my face crumpled and I surrendered, yet again, to tears.

When I finished ugly crying, I gave my face a few minutes to recover, put my coat back on, told Fran I wasn't feeling well, and hurried home. I wanted to fall apart before the kids got home.

Fiona, who had been sleeping on the back of the sofa when I stormed in and sat down, startled at my heaving. She shook her head, stood up, stretched, and then started licking the back of my head. I turned and grabbed her and snuggled her to my chest. She complained but put up with it briefly while I scratched her head. When she'd had enough she leaped away, opening tiny, itchy holes in the skin of my chest. I scrounged in my pockets for a tissue and found a rumpled handkerchief, blew my nose and cried some more. When I'd worn myself out I just flopped over onto the sofa, pulled the *Schitt's Creek* blanket over me, and drifted off into sleep.

The kids were nonplussed to find me lying on the sofa when they got home. I made an excuse about feeling sick after my flu shot and went to my bedroom, where I went back to sleep. When I woke up it was dark out. I got up to pee and went straight back to bed. Kelsey heard me and came in to check on me. I told her she and Eliot should fix dinner for themselves tonight. Then I fretted and tossed and turned for a while, hashing out all the angry things I wanted to say to the PA, to Moose. I thought of texting Jamie but I decided I shouldn't inflict my wretchedness on her.

The next time I woke there was a gray light trying to push its way through the blinds. I rolled over and tried to go back to sleep. I knew I should get up but I just couldn't make myself. It was Saturday, my kids were basically self-sufficient, my job seemed pointless and doomed to failure, my marriage was over and no one would ever love me again. I dreamed I was traveling around Europe with a group of hippies and got my period, leaving blood on the back of my pants, sending me up and down a winding staircase in search of a clean toilet.

"Are you ok, Mom?" Kelsey's voice woke me.

"What time is it?"

"It's eleven o'clock. You never sleep this late."

"Sorry, hon, I'm still not feeling great." That was the truth.

"Do you need anything?"

"No, I'm fine." *Maybe I should have some coffee.* "I think I just need to sleep a little more." She kissed me on the head and took her leave, closing the door gently behind her.

When I woke again it was dark. I didn't know if it was 6 p.m. or midnight. I heard the water running, which probably meant Eliot was in the midst of one of his marathon showers. (I really needed to talk to him about the water bill.) Again I had missed the opportunity to feed my kids. Kelsey came back at some point and asked if I was alive. I apologized and assured her I would be fine. She asked if I had Covid. I said I didn't think so. She went and got the thermometer anyway. No fever. I promised her I was fine and told her I loved her. I got up to pee again, took some ibuprofen for the splitting headache I had from caffeine withdrawal, drank a little water from the tap out of my hand, and went back to bed. I stared at the walls for a while till I went fell into something like sleep. The next morning I was vaguely aware of Kelsey coming in to tell me it was Sunday.

"Mom, please get up," she said, "you're scaring me."

"I will, hon, don't worry." I tried to sound convincing, though I had no intention of getting up. I briefly turned on my phone to check emails and then decided everyone could fuck off. I drifted away again. A few minutes or hours later I heard someone coming up the stairs, walking to my door, and opening it.

"Good morning, starshine," Jamie's voice said. "The earth says hello!" I was instantly comforted and humiliated at the sound of her voice. She took a deep breath. "Whew, it's stuffy in here." I'm sure it smelled disgusting, like sadness and the end of the world. She opened the blinds and the wintery sun streamed in. I hid my head under the covers as I felt her sit down next to me on the bed.

"How'd you get in?" I sounded like my son.

"Kelsey let me in. Actually, she begged me to come over."

"Traitor."

"Are you ill?"

"No, just leave me alone."

"But it's time to get up, gorgeous." She rubbed my back through the blankets. "Your kids need you and the world needs you."

"No they don't!" I whined like a child. "My kids hate me and the world hates me!"

"They don't hate you, Jen," she sighed. "They're teenagers. It's their job to push you away. And it's your job to keep loving them anyway. But for the record," she stage-whispered, "even Eliot looked a little bit concerned." I pulled the blanket down to my nose. She was wearing a beret, the color of which could only be described as raspberry. Her eyes took me in with loving kindness. She put her hand on my forehead. It felt cool and dry. "No fever," she said. "Is anything broken?"

"Yes," I pouted. "All of me is broken."

"Yes, I know," she said soothingly, "you're a wreck, horrible, the worst person who ever lived. But besides that, is there anything *specifically* wrong?"

"No." Then I realized, "I'm hungry and I have a headache. And I'm old and I'll be dead soon."

"Good news, we can fix the hunger and the headache," she said. "But death is a certainty, so you'll just have to deal with that. Come on, get your bad, stinky self in the shower and I'll go make some brunch." She bustled into the bathroom and turned the shower on, clapped her hands and said "Chop chop," then whooshed out the bedroom door.

I pushed my blankets off in a huff and tentatively put my feet on the floor. They felt sore. My hips creaked as I stood. I reached for the ceiling and stretched my aching spine. It kind of hurt but also felt good. I waddled into the bathroom and closed the door. When I took off my pajamas, I looked at my naked body in the mirror—pale, hairy, with all its flab and lumps and curves and droops and spots. The room felt drafty and cold. I sighed and got into the shower. It was hotter than I liked but I left it where Jamie had set it. I shampooed my hair twice before conditioning, just because it felt good, and I scrubbed my body extra vigorously, washing the cobwebs away.

When I was done I stood dripping on the mat and took a clean towel out of the closet. I smelled it first to make sure there was no hint of mildew before rubbing my body with it. I needed to feel my best. There would be a lot of clean up and repair to do that day. I went to my closet and picked out my softest sweatpants, long-sleeved Madison tee, and sweatshirt. I blew my hair dry and went downstairs, feeling almost human.

Jamie had made coffee. She had also cleaned the kitchen, made a pot of oatmeal, cut up an orange and a banana, set the table for two, and turned on some soft jazz. I felt overwhelmed with gratitude and stood dumbly in the doorway. She put her arm around my back and nudged me toward the table. "Come on in, my lovely." She poured coffee, put out two steaming bowls of oatmeal, and nudged a cream pitcher and a small bowl of brown sugar in my direction. "Eat," she said. "You'll feel better."

I did eat, and I did feel better. While I did she nattered contentedly about the things she needed to do at the bookstore that afternoon. She was excited about training a new employee, and about a display table of feminist dystopias inspired by a new bestseller out about a reform school for bad mothers. "Now you," she said. "What's going on?"

"I dunno, everything. Friday was a shitty day." I told her about the doctor and the lawyer and my multiple meltdowns.

"Why didn't you call me Friday?"

"Because I was losing it!"

"It's ok if you lose it, isn't it? You're allowed to have emotions, Jen."

"I know but...you've just been so wonderful ever since we got here and I feel so bad dumping on you. I'm the worst friend! All I've ever given you is my misery and neediness. It's humiliating." Water started leaking from my eyes.

"I get that. You have your pride." She handed me a napkin and gave me a minute to wipe and sniffle. "But also, are you KIDDING me?"

"What?"

"You are so *not* needy! You're one of the most self-sufficient, badass women I've ever known, and you haven't dumped on me at all! And anyway, everyone is needy sometimes. You just didn't know me when I was trying to figure out my sexuality, or when my parents died, or," she waved her hands, "all the things. Trust me, I've been in the depths of despair before. Isn't that what she called it, the 'depths of despair'?" *OMG, did she just make a perfectly-timed Anne of Green Gables reference?*

"You truly are a bosom friend," I said with a sniffle.

She smiled, her eyes twinkling, the parentheses around her narrow mouth becoming deeper. "But not a bosom buddy."

I laughed with relief, my stomach full of oatmeal, my chest full of some positive emotion I couldn't quite name. "Thank you."

"Don't mention it," she said. "That's what bosom friends are for."

Chapter 19

Coming Back from the Edge

In March I tried to move on after my mini-nervous-breakdown. "Nervous breakdown" was a term I hadn't thought of since my 70s childhood, when I heard it on TV—maybe on *Love Boat* or *Dallas*—and it sounded scandalous and mysterious. I was pretty sure today's scientific community recognized no such medical diagnosis, but for whatever reason the term now made perfect sense to me. It made me feel better to give it a name.

In a perfect world, maybe I could have taken a year off to rest, figure things out, and get myself together. But this wasn't a perfect world. I had kids and parents who needed me to function, at least at some basic level, and I was determined to do so. I also had a job to do for a faculty in desperate need of trauma-informed leadership.

The only thing that had changed was that I was finally convinced that I, too, needed help. I had a lead on a therapist, but it would take weeks to get approvals from my health insurance company and find a time when she was free for a new client. So in the meantime, like any good academic, I looked to books for help.

On a Saturday morning, I decided to take a few hours for myself and made a trip to Flyover Pride Books. March hadn't really come in like a lion, as far as I could tell. It was just cold and damp and grey. Patches of crusty, dirty snow lay here and there, making everything ugly. That day was cold, with no detectable signs of spring yet, but I forced myself to walk. I stayed on the far side of the street from the college, lest I run into anyone who might want something from me. When I walked up to Jamie's store I spotted her through the window, making sure all the books on the fiction shelves were flush. I couldn't help smiling. When I walked in and the doorbell jingled, she turned around and smiled back.

"Good day, madam," she said formally, hands together, with a slight bow. "Can I help you find anything?"

"Oh no, thank you," I said, equally formal. "I'm just browsing."

"Well, browse away, my dear. And help yourself to coffee or tea if you'd like, I just made them." She gestured toward a table with two carafes on it, next to a collection of miscellaneous but elegant antique cups sitting upside-down on a tray. I took off my mittens and picked up a tiny flower-shaped cup with pink and white stripes and gold trim.

"Actually," I said in a low voice, swallowing my pride as Jamie poured me some coffee, "do you happen to have any books on menopause?" Her eyes grew wide. "I'm asking for a friend, of course."

"Uh oh," she said, "that sounds serious."

"Yep. It's only recently occurred to me that it might explain a lot about...things." She squeezed my shoulder supportively.

"I've got you, Gen X girlfriend. Come on." She led me toward the back corner opposite the kids' section. There at eye level was a whole shelf of books about women's health, anchored by the ninth edition of *Our Bodies, Ourselves*. "Of course, I can't exactly speak from experience, but a friend recommended this one." She handed me a pink book called *The Menopause Manifesto*. I held it with the thumbs and forefingers of both hands, as if it were dangerous, covered in old lady germs.

"Cripes," I said. "Am I really ready for this time of life?" *You did just say cripes.*

"Ready or not, it's coming for you," she said, matter-of-factly. More softly she added, "Don't worry, sweetie, you'll get through it."

"Easy for you to say," I said with a smirk.

"Yeah, right," she said, "I know absolutely *nothing* about hormones or unwanted chin hairs." That made me feel like an ass and I was afraid I had offended her, but when I looked up she winked at me.

"I'm so sorry," I said with relief, "that was a stupid thing to say."

"It's ok," she said graciously. "But trust me, everyone has body issues at some point. It's just the nature of our bodies to betray us in one way or another. If nothing else, they die." She threw up her hands in resignation.

Since she'd mentioned it, I thought maybe it was time for me to ask her something about her body, though I wasn't sure exactly what or how to ask.

"So… did you… or do you… experience any… issues like… menopause?" It was an ignorant question but, as it happened, I was entirely ignorant. And if Jamie and I were going to be real friends, I would have to trust her enough to take a risk.

"Not really," she shook her head. "I took estrogen for years but it kind of slowed me down and messed with my moods, you know? So now I just take anti-androgens." Holding her hands up to her face she added, "And of course I have a good electrologist."

"I also get the occasional witchy chin hair," I laughed, "but my biggest complaint is how fat I've gotten in the last few years."

"Shh," she said gently, "you really shouldn't say fatphobic things like that about yourself, darling, especially when Kelsey's around. Anyway, I think 'voluptuous' is the term you're looking for." I blushed and scrambled for a way to get back to the subject of her. When did she start wearing dresses? Did she still have testicles? I decided to stick with the topic at hand. "When did you start taking hormones?"

"In my late twenties," she said. "It took me that long to get OK with myself. In college I was still trying to be straight, and then finally senior year I came out as bisexual, but I was still not really OK. Then I went to business school like my dad wanted, and I felt like I had to act 'normal' at work so I self-medicated just to survive. But then *finally*, when I took my head out of my ass, I found my people. I made a queer friend at work, and started going to AA and therapy, and I got sober, hence this section…" She gestured toward a shelf of books on being sober curious and alcohol-free.

"So I was well into my thirties before I really internalized that I didn't have to conform to anybody else's standards."

She scrunched her hair and straightened some books on the shelf. "Then I moved back here to be a death doula for my parents and face all my high school tormentors. Oh and I also gave up being Catholic."

"You're Catholic?"

"I *was* Catholic," she corrected. "Now I go to a Unitarian Church." The doorbell jingled and a group of three customers bustled in.

"To be continued?" I asked.

"Definitely."

I paid the young man at the register for *The Menopause Manifesto*, along with *Why We Can't Sleep*, and one with my favorite title, *What Fresh Hell Is This?* I also got a book called *Boys & Sex* so I could learn about how I had probably already scarred Eliot for life, preventing him from ever having a healthy sexual relationship.

Later that night, after I'd put in a couple of hours at my computer, I found Kelsey half-lying on the sofa under her Taylor Swift blanket watching *Turning Red* and eating candy corn. I grabbed the *Schitt's Creek* blanket (*damn you, algorithm*) and lay down next to her, my head on her hip. "Where'd you get candy corn in March?" I asked, reaching for the bag.

"I found it in the back of the pantry," she said, holding it out to me.

"Ah yes, I probably hid it from myself last fall." I could never resist an open bag of candy corn. I squeezed a single piece between my back teeth, anticipating the satisfying crushing sensation, but these were a bit too crunchy, past their prime. I ate them anyway and immediately started coughing from the sugar. Kelsey patted me on the head, which I found strangely comforting.

"How are you feeling?" I asked.

"Ok," she sighed. "A little crampy."

"Do you have enough pads and everything?" I asked. I could only remember seeing tampons in the bathroom drawer, and she had made it clear that she wanted nothing to do with those.

"Yeah."

"I'll make us some dinner," I said, not moving. That reminded me of my conversation with Jamie. "Hey, sweetie?"

"Hmm?"

"Have I ever made you feel bad about your body?" She didn't reply so I followed up. "I mean, do I bug you about food and weight and stuff like that?" She still didn't reply but I held my tongue and waited.

"Mmm, I guess maybe a little? Like, you always talk about how fat you are, and you always want me to get exercise and eat vegetables. But I don't think you've ever actually told me I'm fat."

"Good, 'cause you're not," I said. Then I hastened to add, "Not that being fat is bad!" *Dammit, Jen.*

"Yeah, but like... it's still kind of a bummer that you always say bad stuff about yourself. 'Cause like..." she trailed off. My eyes felt hot. I took a breath and resisted interrupting. "...you're my mom, you know?"

"Yeah." I had a lump in my throat that wasn't from the candy corn. I squeezed her around her middle. "I'm really sorry, sweets. I'm gonna work on it and try to do better."

The day finally came when I had to get my first mammogram. I was dreading it, but it was long overdue and I knew I was already lucky to have made it to my 50s without any kind of breast cancer. This was part of adulting, so I just

had to do it. I had been instructed not to wear any deodorant that day—apparently it interfered with the imaging—so
I put some in my purse for later. I also threw in a couple of
washcloths in case of inopportune sweating.

I arrived at the hospital, parked in the outpatient section,
and walked into the building. I followed signs to patient
check-in, where I found a large waiting area with a number
of people already there, and a bank of kiosks. I checked in
electronically and sat down to wait. It wasn't long before an
absolutely tiny woman about my age, wearing navy scrubs,
called for Jennifer.

"Hi! I'm Marci," she said when I stood up. "I'll be doing
your mammogram today." I must have looked nervous because she asked, "Is this your first one?"

"Yes. Can you tell?"

"Aw, I understand, but don't worry, it'll be over quickly.
I've been doing this a long time. And these new 3D machines give us a really good picture on the first try, so you
probably won't have to come back." *Yikes.*

"Do people usually have to come back?"

"Well, the old machines used to create some ambiguous pictures that the doctors would usually want to follow up on,
especially for people with dense breasts, but these give a
much better picture. Here we are." She pointed into a dressing room. "Take off everything from the waist up, including
your earrings, and put on the robe there with the opening
in front. Did you put on deodorant this morning?"

"No."

"Good girl. Come on out when you're ready, I'll be right
next door. Bring everything with you."

I did as I was told. The room next door was dimly lit
and relatively warm, compared to the chilly dressing room.

A giant white machine that reminded me of a Kitchen-Aid blender stood to one side. On the other side was a standing desk with a computer monitor on it, and a wall with a window in it that created a small room in the corner.

"You can put your things down on the chair there." I did. "We'll start with your right side, so come on over and pull your right arm out of the robe. Good. Now I'm going to put these on your nipples—" she applied two tiny stickers with metal balls in them "—and then you are gonna come right on up here, as close to the machine as you can get—even closer—and I'm gonna put your breast right here, ok?"

"Ok."

"I'm sorry if my hands are cold." Her tiny, cool hands felt smooth as they grabbed my breast and pulled it up onto a glass plate. She held onto my back to keep me from backing up. "I'm gonna move this up a little bit," the machine buzzed as it adjusted. "How's the height for you?"

"It seems fine."

"OK, now put your cheek up against it, good, and then this is the hard part, but I'll be quick." She turned a crank and another glass plate started smooshing down on my breast. A boob sandwich. "A little more, a little more—are you ok?"

"I guess so?" It was uncomfortable more than painful.

"Ok, good, now don't move, and don't breathe." She darted behind the wall and I heard a tiny buzz. "Ok you can relax." I exhaled.

We did another picture on the right side, except this time I had to lift up my arm so she could smash my boob sideways instead of up and down. Then we did it all over again on the left. While I stood in my robe with my left side hanging out, she looked carefully at the images she had captured.

"Ok, looks good, you're all done."

"Really? That's all?"

"Yep."

"Can you see anything?"

"Oh, I'm sure you want to wait for the doctor to tell you that!"

"Oh right, duh." *Duh?* "How long will that take?"

"Usually just a few days. Do you have any other questions?"

"Nope, I guess not."

"All right, then just put your clothes back on, put your robe in the bin, and you're good to go. You have a great day, all right?"

"All right, you too, thanks."

As promised, I got an electronic notice from my doctor a couple of days later. Apparently, I had "dense breasts" so they couldn't make any promises, but as far as their lawyers would let them say, my breasts looked to be clear of cancer. I felt tremendous relief; I hadn't realized till then that I had been subconsciously worrying about it. *Thank you, universe. I just don't have time for cancer this year.*

Chapter 20

The Terrible, Horrible, No Good, Very Bad Birthday

As if the later winter weather wasn't depressing enough, world news continued to pile on. New wars, old wars, famines, updated climate emergencies. Local news headlines were somewhat more bewildering: "Bobcat Survives Run-In with Car," "Criminology Professor Convicted of Arson," and "Nottawa Township Man Accused of Destroying Bedroom with Chainsaw after Becoming Enraged over Dog Defecating on Floor." *Pure Michigan.*

Work was also making me extra cranky. It was registration season, so all the students were trying to pick their classes for the fall semester, with all the attendant freakouts about not getting all the classes they wanted. Professors were freaking out too, because they had too many or too few advisees to meet with, or the registration software wasn't working properly, or their classes were either too empty or too full. And some were angry because the bookstore manager—simply doing her job—was "nagging" them about ordering all textbooks for their fall classes already, before registration, as federal law required. (In reality, the bookstore was lucky if faculty got their orders in before first-year student move-in day in August.)

A local reporter called the PR office looking for a Russian expert who could comment on current events in Ukraine. The PR intern called me, and I had to tell her we had no such expert on the faculty anymore, since the last one retired in the early aughts and the history department lost that line to the business department. I suggested she contact the adjunct instructor in art history, who specialized in something to do with European Romanticism but who happened to be Ukrainian. Maybe she knew something, or knew someone who knew something.

I made a mental note to talk to the president about this gap in our expertise, and then immediately decided to forget it. I already knew what his response would be. I decided to spend my capital bolstering Environmental Studies instead, which I thought might be an easier sell in a region surrounded by something like twenty percent of the world's fresh water, and was on the minds of Gen Z more broadly.

On March eighth, I turned fifty-two years old. It was my first birthday as a single parent and I woke up determined to have a good day, no matter what.

"Happy birthday, Mom!" Kelsey sang when I came downstairs. She ran to me and gave me a big hug. "Eliot, it's her birthday."

"I know." He frowned, but gave me a one-armed hug. "So, 52, eh? That's really old."

"Why thank you, son."

"We're out of milk," Kelsey said, standing with the fridge door open.

"I'll go to the store later."

"Oh, the car's almost out of gas," Eliot said.

"Well perhaps you should get some on the way to school today."

"There's no time," he whined, "we'll be late."

"On the way home then?" I suggested. "You can get some milk while you're at it."

He rolled his eyes. I knew I would end up filling the tank on the way to the grocery store later. *Happy birthday to me.* I shook it off. Thanks to Covid, I hadn't had a proper birthday in two years, and I wanted to have fun. Jamie and I had plans to celebrate over dinner after work.

"Do you want me to invite anyone else?" she had asked.

I had briefly thought about inviting the Women's Caucus, but decided against it. "Nah, I don't have any other friends here."

"Good, then I'll have you all to myself." That sounded good to me too.

My morning at the office was blessedly quiet, thanks to it being the first day of spring break. This meant that students had forgotten all about college, while faculty and staff had moved their complaints into cyberspace instead of my office.

My email box was full of the usual string of complaints from various folks under my charge. The older librarian hated the new library director's bookless approach to libraries. A young political scientist was angry after finding out his colleague in economics got paid significantly more than he did, despite having been hired the same year. The registrar needed me to sign off on the latest group of academic probationers following mid-terms. I somehow sailed through all these emails—and a few phone calls where I thought it safer not to put anything in writing—with my good mood intact. Everyone seemed satisfied and I felt like an administrative goddess. It was as if I had taken a *Felix Felicis* potion. I was hopeful going into the cabinet meeting.

The cabinet, you see, did not actually get a break. President Festerling was on a fundraising trip to Florida—with his wife and kids—along with the VP for advancement and *his* wife and kids. Both of them joined us by speaker phone while the rest of us sat around the conference table like chumps.

"Greetings, everyone," his voice emerged from the electronic spider on the conference table. "I hope you're having a productive break. Brian and I have already had some very productive meetings here in Tampa." *I'm sure you have.* I had seen a number of his Instagram photos—he and his family smiling in seersucker and sundresses, while we shivered in the slush of a 35-degree heatwave. (Well, everyone except me—my body hadn't gotten the weather report and I was sweating.)

"I know everyone is very busy so I'll get right to the first item on the agenda." He paused, saying something muffled to a child. "Now that the CDC has lifted the mask mandate, we will do the same after break. Tracey and I have already been in touch and she has, I believe, drafted an announcement."

The director of PR nodded silently before remembering he couldn't see her. "That's right," she said, "it's ready to go."

I had of course anticipated this—lots of schools had done so already—so I had planned only the briefest of protests, just to go on record. I had to interrupt because he was already moving on to the second agenda item.

"Sorry, everyone," I said as politely as possible, "Norm, if I may? This is Jen."

After a brief pause (did I hear a sigh?) he said, "Of course, Jennifer, go ahead."

"Thanks," I said. "I'm sorry to always be that person, but I'm wondering if we could consider a modified lifting of the campus mask mandate for the sake of instructors and staff. Of course I leave the matter of student wellness to Kyle," I made eye contact across the table with the VP for student affairs, a millennial with a ponytail and giant hipster beard, "but I would like to propose that we maintain our mask mandate in classrooms for the remainder of the term."

The VP for student affairs looked away. In fact, no one made eye contact except the diversity director, who nodded. My heart was pumping hard and my face flushed. There were going to be huge pit stains on my blouse.

"Yes," came the president's voice, "of course we very much value our instructors and everything they do for our students. Classroom safety is a very important part of what we do here at the College of St. Margaret. Since the CDC has said we can lift mask mandates, we will do so. But of course faculty are welcome to keep wearing masks as they deem appropriate. Kyle and I have already agreed that we no longer need a mask mandate for students." He cleared his throat. "In the interest of your time, let's move on to the second item..."

I'd been dismissed, and tried to slow my breathing as the COO explained why we needed to reassess our tuition and discount rate—raising the former and lowering the latter— in light of the news that an elite little college in Ohio had just announced its tuition was going up to $80,100. The VP of admissions objected strongly, citing how difficult it already was to retain current students and fill next year's incoming class. Our students were not wealthy and would go elsewhere if forced to pay more. This discussion was outside my purview so I bided my time.

Finally, it was my turn on the agenda. I had what I thought was good news and I was excited to share it. I had already discussed it with the VP for advancement before the break, and he had seemed enthusiastic about it too.

"As some of you already know," I began, "a donor approached me directly—an alum from the mid 90s who wants to remain anonymous—who wants to give a large gift for what an endowed chair, the Greta Thunberg Chair of Climate and Environmental Justice. It can be for a scholar in any discipline—so, tree biology, political science, poetry, ethics, or whatever—as long as it's related to Climate and Environmental Justice."

"Do we even have a department of Climate and Environmental Justice?" asked the CFO with a frown.

"No," I said, "it's the name chosen by the donor. It would be a new, inter-disciplinary program headed up by the new chair." The CFO and COO passed a look at each other that I couldn't read. I strived to keep from growing shrill.

"I know we need to be very cautious about donors trying to dictate curriculum, but in this particular case the donor's interests seem to be aligned with the college's liberal arts mission. It's very flexible and a great opportunity, and I believe the faculty would be supportive, since it could potentially go to almost any department." When no one said anything I threw the conversation to the VP for advancement. "Brian, this is a good thing from a fundraising point of view, right?"

"Actually, Jennifer," came Brian's voice from the spider, "I've talked about this with Norm and tested the water with some of our most prominent board members, and I'm afraid this is a no-go." All my sweat turned cold and suddenly I was freezing. "They're really against a chair by that name because it sounds reminiscent of CRT and so forth." *And so forth?* The diversity director looked as if she might vomit. "We're of course very grateful for this donor's wish to be generous, and we appreciate that climate change is a topic worth exploring, but quite frankly we just don't want to be seen as politicizing the curriculum."

"*Politicizing* the curriculum? Are you joking?" I burst out. The spider went silent. Everyone at the table stared at me, aghast. *Walk it back, Jen.* "A topic *worth exploring*? Look around, folks, the curriculum is *already* political. *Every* curriculum is *inherently* political. Liberal arts education used to *explicitly* be about democracy, but now the pre-professional departments have entirely taken over because education is not just for the elites anymore, which is a good thing, of course, but now the zeitgeist would have our graduates serve as cogs in the capitalist system first and foremost, with democracy a distant second. *That's political.*"

I had not walked it back. I could hear the italics in my speech and I was rambling but I couldn't stop.

"We don't teach Russian anymore, or have any historians who know anything about Russia, because no one has cared about Russia for decades. *That's political.* The earth is literally on fire in many places, but we have yet to install a single solar panel on campus or eliminate plastic bottles or switch to alternative energy sources. *That's political.* We're on Potawatomie land but our students are 90% white and we don't have so much as a land acknowledgment plaque *anywhere*, and *meanwhile* we're named after the Catholic patron saint of *expectant mothers* in a country where abortion rights are under attack, but there's no funding for child care or education or maternity leave. That's political. *Everything every single one of us* does is political!"

I was now waving my hands, New Jersey style, and was kind of glad my boss couldn't see.

"*In what universe* do we think a college can isolate itself from politics?" No one answered my rhetorical question. "When you say you don't want to politicize the curriculum, what you're really saying is you don't want to appear to be too *leftist* for your wealthy conservative donors or for the conservative male students you're now desperately trying to recruit."

There was a terrible pause as I finally deflated into my chair. I was shivering and my heart was racing.

"Yes, of course, Jennifer," the boss broke the silence with his predictably bland and patronizing response, "thank you. We all know how important the environment is and of course we appreciate your passion for the liberal arts. Right now, Brian and I are in conversations with various board members and major donors and we're not prepared to take this gift with its current conditions, but it's definitely something to consider going forward."

I shook my head at his Newspeak but held my tongue, lest he decide I was doubleplusungood. *Your kids need health insurance, Jen, and so do you. You can take it up with him privately when he gets back.*

I didn't have to wait till he got back. Before I even walked back to my office, somehow both hot and cold, wet and clammy with old sweat, he texted me an order to call him immediately. (I picked up the pace because I desperately needed a potty break before calling him back.)

"That was quite a performance," he said flatly when I dialed him up.

"I'm sorry, Norm," I sighed. *But are you really?* When he didn't reply right away I added, "I was way out of line. I don't know what got into me today." *Don't you though?*

"It's perfectly appropriate for you to have a contrary opinion, but senior administrators have to set a professional tone for the whole college. You're not faculty anymore. We don't get to shout about things like faculty do."

"I know."

"In case you've forgotten, I was once a philosophy professor."

"Yes, I remember." Something told me he hadn't done much yelling back in those days, either. He was like me. People who yell rarely make the jump to administration because their bosses don't like them.

"I'm well aware," he went on, "of the stress the academic sector is under. I'm also well aware of the tension between *designing* a top-notch education and actually *funding* it. I live that tension every day." He had me there.

"I know, Norm, you're right. You're on the front lines dealing with donors and alumni, and I don't fully understand what that's like. I certainly didn't mean to minimize the difficulty of trying to find enough money to fund the college's mission. I know you and Brian are doing the best you can."

"Thank you. We are."

"I do hope..." *Shut up, Jen, quit while you're ahead!* "...that we can maintain some semblance of academic independence when it comes to rich board members throwing their weight around."

"Yes, and perhaps you could talk to this wealthy environmentalist donor about the name of the endowed chair they're offering to donate." *Touché.*

"I'll see if I can persuade them," I said. I knew the donor was expecting a call back today but I couldn't face it. I needed time to cool down figure out a strategy. *I'll think about that tomorrow,* said the Scarlett O'Hara in my head. Then I felt guilty for quoting a fictional Confederate in my head.

I was completely exhausted at the end of the day and not in the mood for a birthday celebration, however small. I texted Jamie from the office.

<I feel like shit tonight. Rain check?>

<Of course, darling! Is everything ok?>

<Yes, just exhausted. Crappy work day. I'll tell you about it.>

<I'm so sorry! Get some rest. [mended heart emoji] Let me know when you want to reschedule.>

<Let's do something when my kids leave for spring break.> Their break and mine did not match up, so I would soon be home alone for a week while they headed to Costa Rica to see their father and *that woman.*

When I got home that night I just wanted to get out of my work clothes and into my comfies, but that was not to be. Kelsey (in her usual spot on the sofa, texting with friends while watching the new *West Side Story*) reminded me we were out of milk. I put down my briefcase, told her to order a pizza, and walked back out the door. When I turned on the car I was reminded that we were also still out of gas, so I stopped on my way to the grocery store. A small TV screen on the gas pump yelled ads and movie trivia at me while I waited for my tank to fill, arms crossed against the cold. *I miss New Jersey, where self-serve still doesn't exist.*

I hated big box stores (and my kids were apparently incapable of buying things for themselves) so when I got to Meijer I chose a big cart, planning to stock up on multiple gallons of milk and other staples so I wouldn't have to return anytime soon.

When I passed through the bakery, I gave into the urge to buy myself a giant chocolate cake with multicolored sprinkles, and I picked up some chocolate ice cream last thing before the check-out. I remembered a *Hyperbole and a Half* comic that said "CAKE IS THE ONLY THING THAT MATTERS," and right then it felt altogether true. It had been perhaps my shittiest birthday in recent memory, but at least there would be cake.

Chapter 21

Your Fat(phobic) Friend

The following Saturday morning Jamie and I drove the kids to the Gerald R. Ford International Airport, from whence they would fly to Costa Rica via Dallas. They hadn't flown without me before, much less internationally, so I went overboard with both verbal and written instructions, eliciting many eye rolls and exasperated exhales. After dropping them off, Jamie and I went to spend the day in "the city," which now meant Grand Rapids instead of Manhattan. *One takes what one can get.*

We went first to see the earliest possible matinée of *Umma,* not because we loved horror but because we loved Sandra Oh (especially since she had recently brought the plight of humanist academic administrators to life as *The Chair* on Netflix). Then we went to find Indian food for lunch, since such cuisine was non-existent around St. Jutta. The movie was fair, but the food was delicious. We gorged ourselves on medium spicy dishes in multiple colors as

Guru Nanak and the other human gurus looked down upon us serenely from the wall.

After lunch we went to visit an independent bookstore, the owners of which Jamie knew casually through unofficial Michigan bookstore owners' networks. The store was quite unlike Jamie's, immaculate and bright, more Scandi minimalism than girlish whimsy. It smelled like fresh paint, and the door was accompanied by an electronic beep rather than jingling bells. The only bit of clutter I noticed was an elderly-looking cat sleeping in a bed next on the check-out desk.

"Helloooo," Jamie called when we entered.

"Oh hey, Jamie!" said a fit-looking bald man in a flannel shirt, with a dark lumberjack beard. He was shelving books in Religion and Spirituality, between Philosophy and Travel. They greeted each other with cheek kisses. "What brings you here?"

"Just out for a day of fun with my bestie." *I'm her bestie?* "Jeff, I'd like you to meet Jen."

"Nice to meet you," he said shaking my hand firmly. "Scott," he called to the back of the store.

"What?" came a voice from behind sci-fi.

"Come here, look who it is." A petite man with curly blond hair, giant black glasses, and a V-neck cashmere sweater appeared out of the sci-fi section. Like Scott, he looked forty-ish. More greetings and kisses and introductions ensued.

"This is such a lovely shop," I said, trying to keep them talking. "How long have you had it?"

"Oh, we probably started around the same time as Jamie." Scott said. He looked at her and she nodded. "We got sick of the banking industry and decided to do something more constructive with what was left of our lives. The store is kind of my baby, and Jeff helps out. He's doing grad school for his midlife crisis."

"Oh really?" Grad school always piqued my interest. "What are you studying?"

"It's a low-residency Master of Divinity."

"How fascinating! Where?"

"Naropa University. It's just for fun," he added bashfully. "I'm not planning to become a religious leader or anything."

"Studying for fun is the best," I said.

"Jen's an Italian scholar and a higher ed administrator," Jamie offered.

"Ugh, then I'll bet you're often stuck in the spreadsheets like me," said Scott. "Hey, let's get out of here and go for a drink." Jamie and I looked at each other. "I mean after you have time to browse, of course."

"That sounds great," I said, having discerned that Jamie's expression meant she was up for it but wanted to make sure I was too.

We hung out and chatted and browsed for more than an hour. I was relieved when my phone whistled with a text from Kelsey, who had arrived in Dallas and said everything was going ok so far. When two college students came in for their shift, Jeff and Scott walked us to a Belgian-themed brewery down the street (one of many breweries in Grand Rapids, which called itself "Beer City USA"). It was charming, dark and high-ceilinged, in what looked to be an old chapel. Jamie offered to drive us home in my car so I could enjoy a flight of five tiny beers.

"So what brought you to Michigan?" Jeff asked.

"I got a job," I shrugged. "In academia you pretty much go anywhere you can get a full-time job with benefits."

"What's the job?" Scott asked. I spent the next few minutes trying to explain what a "provost" was, trying to explain the byzantine structures of higher ed administration and community governance, trying to explain how no one actually had any authority to do anything, except the president, and even he answered to the trustees, none of whom actually worked in higher education. The men across from me looked more and more bemused as I went on.

"Jeez, no wonder higher education is crumbling," Scott said when I finally came up for air.

"Hon," Jeff said, alarmed.

"What?" Scott said defensively. "Every day I read a new article about it. I'm sure she's well aware."

"Yeah, it's pretty rough. But," I felt obligated to add, "I am still a true believer in liberal arts education. It's definitely not cheap or efficient, but it's one of the best ways to get adults to genuinely expand their minds and see things in a new way. I mean most people would otherwise never talk to anyone they don't already like, or read a book they don't already want to agree with, you know?"

They nodded. Jamie watched me with an admiring smile, her laugh lines on full display. My face and chest were warm, whether from beer or a hot flash or just the thrill of talking to people about stuff I cared about.

"It's a real conundrum," I went on. "People who go into academia are almost by definition bad at business and administration. I mean, I studied Italian Renaissance literature! What do I know about managerial accounting?"

Jeff looked at Scott. "Babe, maybe you should start a higher ed side hustle." They laughed.

"So yeah," my thoughts were flooding out of me, "it's really hard to find someone who really *gets* the mission of higher education, but is also good at leading… and problem solving and trouble shooting and organizing and communication and marketing and fundraising and all the things that have to happen for a college to survive. Not to mention coaching athletics and mental health counseling and real estate management.

"So then you have to hire all these extra people who aren't there to teach classes, but they are absolutely necessary to keeping the place running. I mean students wouldn't even come if they couldn't play baseball or whatever, or join fraternities and have a social life. And they also won't come unless they can major in something 'useful' that makes their parents happy, like nursing or business or pre-med, and of course *those* majors are the hardest and most expensive to staff. So then colleges keep chopping off parts of our bodies, like Italian, that aren't the expensive parts but they just seem like parts no one will miss."

I suddenly felt choked up and willed myself not to cry.

"But then that still doesn't really solve the problem, because we still can't find enough people to teach nursing or accounting, or people who want to move to rural Michigan for what little we can afford to pay them. So then poor towns like St. Jutta live under the constant threat of their largest local employer going belly-up, which would be absolutely terrible for the town, even though the locals complain about the college and the students and the liberal snowflakes trying to indoctrinate the youth."

I cut myself off there, already feeling it was too late. My face had gone from warm to burning hot.

"Wow," Scott said. "That's a lot."

"Yeah," Jeff added. "I had no idea it was that bad."

Jamie put her arm around my shoulders and interjected, "So now you can see why she's my new bestie!" We all laughed. We raised our pints or our sparkling water or our tiny glass and we toasted to tilting at windmills until we couldn't tilt anymore. Then I excused myself to go to the bathroom, where I stuffed paper towels under my soaking wet boobs. I checked myself out in the mirror to make sure my scarf hid the bulges.

As we drove home through dusky farmland, keeping our eyes open for deer, I apologized to Jamie for being such a downer. "I hope I didn't embarrass you in front of your friends."

"Oh darling, never apologize for speaking your truth," she said. "And they're not really my friends, they're just colleagues." She thought for a second. "But who knows? Maybe after tonight we'll be friends, now that you let your freak flag fly." She put her hand on top of mine on my knee. My stomach fell down into my groin. "Anyway you never have to be embarrassed around me."

I actually believed her. Nothing seemed to fluster her. She always seemed composed, quick to smile, slow to anger. In any other context I would have envied her, but something about Jamie elicited admiration rather than envy. I thought of her next-door neighbor's Trump sign.

"How can you stand living in St. Jutta, with all the people who used to be mean to you, and the conservatives judging you?"

She shrugged, her eyes on the road. "I don't know. I just don't care anymore, I guess. I spent my whole childhood and adolescence and young adulthood trying to be a certain way and caring about what other people thought of me. Little by little I figured some things out, and then at some point I had an epiphany that I could just...*not care.* I still care about people, but only about stuff that matters." She thought for a moment. "I mean, it certainly doesn't make me *happy* to know that some people hate the fact that I exist. But I also don't feel responsible for changing them, you know? If they want to be upset about my clothing or my sex life that's on them."

Please tell me more about your sex life, I wanted to say.

"Anyway," she smiled, "corrupting the youth is *your* job."

"That's amazing," I said. "I've always been obsessed with what people think—if I'm hurting their feelings, or they think I'm fat or ugly, or they don't think I'm smart or can't do my job well, or..." I sighed. "It's pathetic, isn't it? I mean, I'm over 50 now! When do I get to start not giving a fuck and just enjoy being an adult?"

"Habit energy is very hard to break," Jamie said. "Don't be too hard on yourself. You're doing the best you can, which is pretty damn good, by the way."

"Let's talk about something other than my lifelong psychoses," I said. "Let's talk about YOUR lifelong psychoses!"

"Oh honey, don't get me started. I could fill a book about that, but life's too short."

Our belated birthday date was not yet over. Back in St. Jutta, we had dinner at the Dragon's Lair. When we walked in, I felt immediately too hot and kind of queasy from the odd smells wafting about. The place was surprisingly full. We were seated at a tall, two-person table just past the bar. I ordered something called a honey badger because it made me laugh (who cares that it was so 2015?), and Jamie ordered mint and cucumber mocktail.

"To your new year," Jamie toasted.

"Thank you!" I clinked. I was still a little buzzed from my tiny beers, so after a sip of my cocktail I said, "I don't mean this to sound cheesy, but, I just feel so lucky to have met you this year, Jamie. I have no idea where I would be if I hadn't!"

"Likewise, darling!" she replied.

"I guess buying a house across the street from you is one last thing I can thank Moose for."

"Oh I wouldn't go that far," she said with a sly smile. "Let's thank the universe instead, shall we?"

The door opened and in came the Women's Caucus. A whoosh of cold air reached us a moment later. They were all carrying gift bags and Joanne was wearing a witch's hat. This was weird, given that we were months past Halloween. The server came with our food and we ordered another round of drinks. Then I excused myself to go to the toilet.

On the way back I passed the Women's Caucus table. I noticed they sat in the same pattern they sat in at the diner. "Good evening, all," I said, as casually as I could, suddenly conscious that seeing me might dampen their mood. "How's everyone doing?"

Vivian answered, "We're having a croning celebration in honor of Joanne's hysterectomy."

"A croning celebration?"

"It's all the rage among feminist witches," said Elaine. "Cronehood is the final stage in a woman's life, after maiden and mother, when she's no longer in the birthing stage."

"I haven't birthed a child in twenty years," Joanne said gleefully, "but whatever!"

"I skipped mother altogether and just went from maiden to crone," added Barbara.

"Joanne is now joining those of us in the senior matriarchy of the tribe," said Vivian.

"Congratulations," I said lamely. "When was your surgery?" It was weird that I didn't know.

"Two weeks ago."

My mouth dropped open. "And you're already up and about?" I remembered my aunt being in bed for weeks.

"Oh yeah," she said with a little wave, "it's no big deal anymore. They just go in through your belly button."

"Well then, great!"

"Do you want to join us?" She gestured politely to the end of the table.

"No thanks," I said, "I'm here with a friend." They all stretched their necks to see who I was with. "I just came over to say hello—and to find out about the hat."

"Oh, that's Jamie from the bookstore," Barb said, waving. Jamie waved back. Somehow she managed to look both cute and elegant at the same time. I felt proud to be sitting with her. I went back to the table where Jamie and I shared a dinner of bacon-covered brussels sprouts, fish and chips, and a piece of cheesecake. The food was mediocre at best, but being with Jamie made it fun anyway.

The last event in our all-day belated birthday extravaganza was the college's dance concert. I was already exhausted and would have much preferred to be at home on the couch, but felt I professionally obligated to attend, in part because tenure and promotion decisions for instructors depended on their production of artistic works. Jamie, on the other hand, went willingly and enthusiastically because she used to dance in college.

"I was almost always the only man around, surrounded by women," she said wistfully, as we walked toward campus.

"It was heaven. Or it would have been, if I didn't have to always dance the man's part." She was joking, but it struck me that it probably hadn't been funny at the time.

"That must have been really hard."

"Yeah, it was sometimes. But at least there were no other dudes around. It gave me a safe space to experiment." After a few moments she said, "I wonder how all those women are. Some of them were really great people. My thirtieth reunion is coming up; maybe I should go."

"Have you ever been back to Oberlin for a reunion?"

"Nope. I never even considered it. But I think I might be ready now." She looked surprised at herself. "Huh! Look at me, I'm growing up!"

"Brava!" I said.

The theater was about half full and, to my relief, not too hot. I put on a mask as we walked in. We hung our coats in the coat room, presented our tickets, and a student usher led us to seats on one of the inner aisles about halfway down, where I hoped people would see me and give me credit for being an engaged provost. I turned on my phone flashlight and pulled out my reading glasses so I could peruse the program.

"You look so cute in those," Jamie said.

"Thanks. I never needed them till a couple of years ago."

"They make you look *extra* smart." She bumped her shoulder into mine.

"Do you ever wear glasses?" I asked.

"Not anymore. I used to wear really thick glasses but I had Lasix years ago when I stopped drinking and started running. I'm sure I'll need readers eventually and I can't wait. I'm gonna get one of those cool old lady chains and wear them around my neck."

The lights went down and the concert started. I turned off my phone. The chair of the department (also the only full-time faculty member in the dance and theater department) had choreographed a witty piece that sometimes seemed like ballet, other times modern, sometimes even folkish, with a little tap dance thrown in for good measure. I wasn't sure what it meant but I liked it.

There was another piece by a part-time adjunct instructor called *Fragmented, Not Yet Defragmented*, which started out with dancers striking poses in groups under spotlights; then everything went dark, and when the spotlights came back up they were in a different spot on the stage, in a different pose. Eventually there were lots of them in various flesh-toned leotards that blended in with their skins, and paper-thin skirts that suggested broken glass. Sometimes they were dancing in sets, sometimes alone; they reached for the sky and crashed to the ground; they bounced in place with their arms flailing like marionettes, and sailed on and off stage as if someone were chasing them.

The dance that struck me most was by another part-time adjunct from Grand Rapids. She had her dancers wearing all-black onesies with blue surgical masks everywhere—on their elbows and knees, around their waists like belts, on their shins like shin-guards. On their faces they had masks too, but they were full-face masks made of flowers. The effect was kind of creepy, like Michael Myers had gotten hold of a hot glue gun and joined up with Mummenschanz. I was captivated as they crept sideways like bugs across the floor. Instead of music, the "dance" was set to sounds of protest marches in different languages. The dancers went in and out of formation. I had really no idea what it was trying to say but I loved it. It made me feel something that was hard to name—exhilaration, maybe, or longing. Or something like joy.

After the show I ran to the restroom. I checked my phone while sitting on the toilet and saw that Moose had texted to let me know he had the kids. That came as a relief. While washing my hands I looked in the mirror and saw an unremarkable middle-aged woman. I couldn't help thinking about all the bodies I had just seen. Most of the student performers were shaped like you'd expect dancers to be shaped: long and lean, with tiny butts and tiny boobs. But there were a handful of bigger women in the mix, whom I found both horrifying and fascinating. In a million years, I couldn't imagine putting my body on a stage in a leotard for people to look at. *I can hardly stand looking at myself.*

When I came out of the bathroom, Jamie was talking to Alain, the department chair. They knew each other from St. Jutta's tiny queer community, which just happened to overlap with its tiny arts community. I congratulated Alain on the concert and on his piece in particular.

"Thanks," he said modestly. "I've been teaching so much dance history lately that it's working its way into my chore-ography. Jamie, you probably recognized Ballanchine? And Martha Graham?"

"Yes, and Alvin Ailey, too, right?"

"Yes!" Alain seemed gratified that at least someone had picked up on his inside jokes. They promised to get to-gether soon and Jamie and I headed out of the crowded lobby. We had left the car near the restaurant so we locked arms as we walked the few blocks back toward downtown. She was cold, but I left my coat unzipped so I could cool off my overheated core.

"That was fabulous," she said. "I love seeing the arts alive and well, especially when the rest of the world is a dumpster fire. They really brought it tonight, the choreographers and the dancers."

"Totally." I wasn't sure what to say that wouldn't betray my ignorance about dance, so instead I said something even worse. "I was so impressed with all the performers, especially the bigger ones."

"What do you mean?"

"I mean, some of those women were...you know, far from thin, but they could really dance, despite their size. I really admire that they're willing to put their bodies on stage where everyone can see them. I could never do that." Jamie pulled her arm out of mine and stopped walking.

"Oh my god, Jen." She grimaced and covered her eyes with her hands. Her nails sparkled with the glittery gold polish I had given her for Christmas.

"What?" I asked. She just groaned. "What?" I said again, now alarmed.

"Why are you like this?" She let her hands fall and looked me straight in the eyes. My stomach lurched.

"Like what?"

"You can just be...so shallow sometimes." That was like a punch in the chest.

"I am *not* shallow," I said, sounding like Kelsey when Eliot was giving her a hard time. "I was complimenting them!"

"But do you even hear yourself? You are fifty-two years old and a feminist with a Ph.D. and the mother of a daughter and you're literally commenting on other women's body sizes."

"I'm sorry!" I protested. "Anyway *you* have no idea what it's like to grow up as a girl in this culture, where you can never look good enough no matter how hard you try, no matter how many diets you go on and how much makeup you buy. I can't help the stupid thoughts that pop into my head!" I was on the verge of tears.

"Yes, I know," she threw up her hands, exasperated, "I *know* you struggle with body image, and I *know* you're not personally responsible for the beauty myth. But when are you going to get over it? It's time to grow up!" She took my hands, softening her voice. "You're an educator and a mom, Jen. There are kids you're passing this onto now."

I jerked my hands away. "Well you don't know anything about being a mom, either, so how about you quit judging me?" I started storming toward the car.

"Jen—"

I turned back. "Do you want a ride home or not?" She just looked at me, her breath coming out in visible puffs under the streetlight.

"I think I'll walk," she said, now sounding angry herself. She turned away, but before leaving she turned back and pointed a finger at me. "And by the way, that's some TERF-level shit you just spouted." Her boots clip-clopped away into the darkness.

I walked off in the opposite direction, furious. *How dare she judge me?* I turned through the alley and took the back way to my car so I wouldn't run into anyone. The wind felt sharp on my cheeks. My heart was racing and I felt tears on my cheeks. By the time I got to my car, my fury had turned on me. *Am I really shallow? Am I a TERF?* I was ashamed of my thoughts; ashamed Jamie had noticed them and ashamed that I had yelled at her when she was just being a friend to me.

I drove home but hadn't quite cooled down by the time I arrived, so I walked around the block. Moose used to tell me I was fat-phobic too, though not in so many words. In fact, the fatter I had gotten myself in middle age, the less forgiving I had become about other people's fat. It had been easier to be magnanimous back when I thought I'd never be one of "them." Now when I looked at myself, especially in pictures, I saw someone I hardly recognized. A fat old white lady, the sort no one notices unless for purposes of ridicule.

When I got home, Fiona was sitting in the front window. I had completely forgotten about her. She got up when she saw me coming and met me at the door. She had been alone all day and demanded to be scratched. I obliged her, grateful for someone who couldn't hear my stupid thoughts. She followed me upstairs where I brushed my teeth, changed into pajamas, glanced at my emails, and determined there was nothing that couldn't wait till tomorrow (or until 3:00 a.m. when I woke up in a sweat and couldn't go back to sleep).

Before turning out the light I texted Jamie. It took me several tries to compose a text before I hit send.

<I'm so sorry. You're right about everything.>

<You are forgiven.> came a reply after an agonizing ten minutes. Relief flooded my chest.

<Can we please talk tomorrow?> I asked.

<Yes, please.>

<Thank you. And thank you for a wonderful day. Sleep well.>

She didn't reply. I would not sleep well, but at least my tossing and turning would be free from dread that I'd just lost my new best friend.

That night I dragged my CPAP out from the back of the closet, dusted it off, and put it on. I had read in one of my books that many women start snoring or get sleep apnea during menopause, because lower levels of progesterone cause the tissues in our airways to "relax." Not breathing well contributes to not sleeping well, which aggravates brain fog and moodiness. Lying there with an oxygen tube to my nose felt like acknowledging defeat—to Moose, to the mean doctor, and to the universe, all of whom seemed to be constantly reminding me of how close I was to death. But at that point I needed all the help I could get.

Early the next morning, I drove down to the Mennonite bakery right when it opened at 7:00 and bought a dozen cinnamon-sugar doughnuts. I brought them straight to Jamie's and rang the doorbell. An early riser, she opened her front door and stood for a moment, looking at me from behind the glass storm door with an expression I couldn't read. She was in a state I rarely caught her in—except when I happened to see her on the street from a distance, coming back from her early morning run—a nondescript fleece and leggings, no makeup, hair up. *A dude with a man bun*, I recalled her saying, back when I hardly knew her.

She was still stunning.

"We don't want any," she said through the door. A dad joke. A good sign. Deirdre, whom I hadn't noticed till then, let out a little yap at her feet.

"But they're from the Mennonites," I pleaded. She pursed her lips and rolled her eyes.

"Ugh, fine, come in." She picked up Deirdre, turned her back, and let me open the storm door myself.

I followed her through the dim living room and dining room, where every surface was covered in something cool that I wanted to stop and look at. I lingered for a few seconds over an abstract stained-glass map of the Great Lakes that was lit up from behind, but then remembered I was on a mission. I went into the kitchen, where the island was lit by warm pendant lights shaped like ice cubes. She was sitting on a tall stool, with a cup of tea and the New Yorker crossword puzzle. I noticed she used a pen. She had put Deirdre down and the ugly-cute creature came over and sniffed my shins.

"That stained glass is really cool," I pointed toward the dining room.

"A friend made it."

"I just realized I've only been inside your house once before."

"Well, here it is." She made a half-hearted *ta-da* gesture.

"You always come to us."

"Yeah, well, you have kids. It's easier for you." She leaned her elbows back on the island, head in her hands. I put the box down and sat next to her.

"Jamie."

"What," she said without moving.

"Jamie."

She sighed and finally looked at me. Her eyes were puffy and she wore the barest hint of a sad smile that broke my heart. "What, Jen?"

I wanted badly to hold her but restrained myself. "I'm so, so sorry."

"I know you are. It's all right."

"It's not all right," I said. "Nothing about it is all right. I'm in a very bad place right now, for a million reasons, and

I can't escape my own self-loathing, especially about my aging body, which I then project onto other people. And I *am* fat-phobic, and it's horrible, and I know it, and all you did was tell me the truth about it.

"And then I got defensive and took it out on you and said something hurtful and stupid and TERF-y, even though I know—I know—you've had to work so hard to learn to love yourself and your body, and to struggle to get to such a good place and become your true self. But honestly, I sometimes forget you went through all that because I didn't know you till you were already amazing."

"I was always amazing, darling," she said, shaking her adorable forelock out of her eyes, "I just didn't know it, same as you."

"It's not your fault I'm this way and I haven't done the work yet."

"No, but you're doing it now, right?"

"I'm trying."

"That's enough for me."

"I'm gonna try harder," I said, putting my hand on hers.

"I know you are."

"I'm sorry again."

"I forgive you again." She put her other hand on mine.

"Really?" I put my other hand on hers.

"Really."

"Thank you."

"You're welcome." There was a moment of silent electricity between us before she said, "Now let's house those doughnuts before I have to get ready for work."

When I got home later that morning, I thought about what "doing the work" would mean for me. When had I become so obsessed with appearances? Most of my life I'd had it easy—white privilege, ableist privilege, straight-size privilege—and I had lived in relative peace with myself and my body. Puberty hadn't hit me too hard; I was neither the first nor the last girl to get boobs, and when I did get them they weren't too big or too small. When my period arrived, it never gave me terrible cramps or anything like that. And even though I'd never been a knockout, I'd always felt attractive enough for my purposes. There were of course some things about my body I'd always wished were otherwise, but I just didn't dwell on them.

Perimenopause, I realized, was something else altogether. It was the first time I'd ever felt at war with my body. It wasn't just the hot flashes and peeing and weight gain, which were bad enough. But I sometimes felt that the mood swings and insomnia were actually going to kill me prematurely. Being suddenly single and surrounded by new people hadn't helped because I was constantly aware of making first impressions, measuring myself against what I imagined they saw in me.

But for the first time, I realized that my bodily discomfort was an occasion for solidarity with my fellow mortals —an opportunity to try to better understand people who struggled with their bodies, or wished for different ones. To see myself among them, and think of them—and myself— with compassion instead of judgment.

I was still thinking about this on Monday morning when I passed St. Margaret on the way to the office. She looked disappointed in me, as if she agreed with Jamie that I was shallow. *Easy for you to judge, permanently svelte in your marble robes.* I wondered if women in her day worried about staying young and thin as much as we did, or if most of them just felt lucky to make it to thirty without starving or dying in childbirth or being martyred for their religious convictions. *Try that, Jen. Just be grateful to live another day, even in this foreign-feeling body.* It wasn't a long-term solution, but it would have to do for now.

Finally, to Therapy

On the second weekend of my kids' spring break, I made a quick trip to NJ to lay eyes on my folks and make sure they were ok. Months had already flown by since I'd seen them at Christmas. I was relieved that they seemed pretty stable for the moment, with no immediate crises. I hoped they could hold on like that for a few more years till I could get my kids launched.

Speaking of my kids, I timed my return trip to Grand Rapids to coincide with their return flight from Costa Rica, where apparently they'd had a fantastic time. (Or rather, Kelsey had a fantastic time; Eliot said it was fine.) The baby—a girl if the ultrasound could be trusted—was due any day and Kelsey was disappointed she hadn't arrived during their visit. She kept checking her texts to see if she'd heard any news from Moose. *You'll get through this, Jen. Just keep moving.*

At the spring equinox, I finally had my first therapy session. I had chosen someone based in Kalamazoo so as to avoid uncomfortable accidental run-ins, and I had double-checked to make sure she wasn't married or otherwise closely connected to anyone who worked at the college. She had suggested that we meet in person at least the first time, if we were both vaccinated and boosted (we were), and then after that we could meet virtually.

The drive was pretty long, and I was kind of looking forward to having some time to listen to the radio and catch up on the news. Russia was still pummeling Ukraine, and the confirmation hearings for a new Supreme Court justice had begun. The first Black woman to be appointed was being forced to listen and respond politely as mostly old, white, male members of the Senate Judiciary Committee mansplained, cast aspersions upon, and even yelled about her judicial record, asking questions that were often unworthy of even an undergraduate 101 classroom. I listened as long as I could, but I shut it off when a hot rock of pain developed in my chest as one of the senators gleefully read out accounts of child pornography.

I would have to drive alone with my own thoughts, most of which were about my bladder.

I had been to Kalamazoo only once before, at what was probably Michigan's best small liberal arts college, for an athletics meeting among administrators in our conference. This time I looked more closely. It was a city that had clearly seen better days, with lots of old buildings that used to be beautiful and were now decrepit, intermingled with some uninspired architecture from the 60s and 70s. But there were also signs of people making an effort—several new-looking brew pubs and restaurants, little museums, a renovated hotel. *You know gentrification is problematic, right?*, my inner Eliot reminded me.

"I wish you well, Kalamazoo," I said out loud.

The therapist's office was in a residential neighborhood a few blocks from downtown, on a street with lots of tall, thick trees. I turned into the driveway of a blue and green Victorian. A sign to the left of the detached garage said "Parking" and, when I obeyed, I saw another sign posted on the house that said "Office," with an arrow pointing around back. I was feeling nervous and checked my face and hair in the rear-view mirror. *What if she doesn't like me? What if she decides I'm hopeless?*

I walked up to a homey but professional looking door with a window that said, in painted letters, NANCY VAN-DEVENTER, MA, MDIV, LMFT. There was no doorbell so I knocked on the wood and soon saw someone coming. A very short, grey-haired woman with crinkly eyes and a big smile answered the door and greeted me warmly as she invited me inside. I loved her immediately and grew even more desperate for her to like me. I self-consciously asked for the bathroom and she non-judgmentally pointed the way.

When I came out, she invited me into a comfortable-looking room with low lighting, chock full of friendly clutter. Some of it was basic grandma kitsch—pottery tchotchkes shaped by tiny hands in art class, a stick figure portrait that said "To Grammy love Jake," a framed collage of family photos. Some of the other clutter suggested she was perhaps ahead of her time for a Baby Boomer, but just slightly cringey by today's standards—masks and baskets and textiles from indigenous cultures I couldn't identify that felt vaguely colonialist. She saw me looking.

"Have you been to West Africa?" I hadn't. "Everything on that wall is from Benin. I was in the Peace Corps there back in the early 90s. It's an amazing place."

I felt ashamed for getting caught being judgmental. I wasn't even sure where Benin was. (Besides Nigeria and South Africa, I pretty much only knew the African countries that had previously been colonized by Italians.) I made a mental note to look it up on a map later.

The room was surprisingly spacious, with high ceilings and large windows on the two corner walls. Both were covered by sheer curtains, I assumed for privacy, but they let some natural light in. A sturdy antique desk sat in front of one window, and small armchair was positioned in front of the other. On a small circular coffee table, a box of tissues and a dusty bowl of potpourri, possibly from the 1980s, kept each other company. Nancy closed the door behind me, grabbed a notepad and pen from the desk, and invited me to sit on the love seat next to the door. She sat down in the armchair, crossed her legs, laid her hands in her lap, and let out an audible exhale, as if centering herself. She blinked and smiled.

"Welcome, Jennifer."

"Thanks."

"I'm glad you're here."

"Thanks, I'm...glad to be here?" *Why did I say that? Because you're always a good girl that's why.* "Actually that's not true. I'm not really glad to be here, I'm only here because my life is falling apart and I'm out of ideas."

"Why don't we start with you telling me a bit about how your life is falling apart."

"Um, ok, but I'll have to talk quickly to fit it all in in an hour," I laughed. She smiled kindly but said nothing. "I'm not sure where to start." My brain rushed through the last few disastrous months of my life. When I finally opened my mouth things started pouring out. I told her my husband had left me for a younger woman and fled the country, just before I dragged my kids to Michigan and abandoned my elderly parents right when they needed me most.

I told her how I'd started a new job where success seemed impossible and I couldn't make friends, given my position. I told her about feeling trapped financially and professionally because I'd never find another academic job if I quit this one, and I had no other way to support myself and my kids.

I told her how much my son hated me and how I could see him grieving, both for the earth and his missing father, and I couldn't help, but at least he had a girlfriend. I told her how I was probably ruining my daughter in real time with all my dysfunction, that she was being brave and cheerful for my sake to compensate for her brother's dickishness, even though she was in the thick of puberty and she, too, needed freedom to be a normal cranky teenager.

]I told her about hating my aging body—about my new disastrous clumsiness, gaining weight, not sleeping, developing wrinkles and sagging and hairs and moles, not being able to reliably control my bladder or sometimes my bowels, about how everything just seemed to hurt all the time for no reason. I told her I probably had a brain tumor that was making me behave erratically. I told her about the horrible doctor visit and Moose's new baby and my mini-nervous breakdown.

Finally, I told her about how I missed my old friends and thought Jamie was going to be my new best friend until I alienated her with my immaturity and also I might be a little bit in love with her.

Somewhere amid the flood of words I had started ugly crying, but I didn't notice until I finally stopped talking and saw a pile of used tissues on the sofa next to me.

"And all I do is cry anymore!" I nearly shouted.

I grabbed three more tissues in rapid succession and carelessly wiped my eyes with them before blowing my nose loudly. We sat silently for a few moments while I took big, heaving breaths, the way I used to cry when I was a kid.

Through all of that she had said nothing, not interrupting once, even to ask a clarifying question. Nor had she taken any notes. She just watched me attentively, occasionally nodding or making a quiet "Mmm." When I finally dared to look up at her again she was looking back at me, waiting for me to be ready. Then she asked, "How do you feel after saying all that?"

I scoffed. "I don't know, relieved I guess." I picked up my hands and flopped them back in my lap. "And a little gross."

"What does that feel like in your body? Where is the relief?" I thought that was a weird question but I considered it, mentally scanning my body for sensations.

"Um, mostly here I think?" I put my hand on my chest. She nodded but said nothing. "And maybe also in my face?" My fingertips floated up to my cheekbones.

"You've been holding onto all that tension and grief in your chest and in your face," she repeated.

"Yeah." I sniffed and thought some more. "Also in my shoulders, like in the middle of them," my left hand rubbed behind my right shoulder, "kind of on the back side of where my chest has been hurting."

"Let's take another moment to pay attention to how your body feels. And try leaving a hand on your chest." I did as instructed. I took a few shallow breaths and then eventually one big one.

"That's a big sigh," she said. "What does it feel like now?"

"Like a weight has been lifted off me?" That seemed too cliché to be the right answer, but it was actually true for the moment.

She nodded. "And what about your face? You said your face felt relieved."

"Around my cheekbones. It felt like I'd been holding my face in a weird position for a long time and finally relaxed."

"Good," she said. "So this is an exercise you can do on your own now and then, when you're feeling stressed. You can take a few minutes to scan your body, maybe especially paying attention to your chest and shoulders and your face, and see if you can breathe into them, or even put your hands on them until they relax."

I nodded. I hated thinking about my body, but I always liked being given a clear assignment that could be checked off a list.

"So we have about fifteen minutes left," she said. "Where would you like to go from here right now?" I wasn't sure, but she didn't fill in the silence for me.

"I guess we could talk about Moose. He makes me feel furious and guilty at the same time."

"Tell me more about that."

"Well obviously I'm pissed off that he left me, and that he left the kids at the hardest possible time in their lives. And I'm doing a terrible job at single parenting, and now he'll always be perfect in their minds and I'll just be the parent they were stuck with when the good parent disappeared. And meanwhile *my* parents are getting to be like kids too, but not having my partner around means I can't go visit them very often. Plus seeing my parents get old reminds me that I'm getting old, and now I'm growing old all alone instead of with the person who was supposed to be there for me."

"So you're feeling resentful about him leaving at this very difficult season of life."

"We were so close to having an empty nest!" I whined. "And like, getting to that part of life that's supposed to be fun again, you know? The part that's the payoff for all the hard stuff we had to do."

"You feel abandoned and robbed of getting to enjoy the fruits of your labor."

"Yeah. But I'm also pissed at *myself* for being so... so..." I hoped she would fill in the blank but she didn't. "For not seeing it coming. And now for not being up to the task, I guess? I'm not doing *anything* well. Not one thing—not work, not parenting, not even being a good friend. I'm just this quivering pile of unmet needs, and I'm still trying to keep doing all the stuff I used to do when most of my needs were met."

"Having a partner was important to your needs being met," she said.

It seemed obvious now. I nodded.

"I always thought we had a good partnership. He wasn't perfect but neither was I. We both did different stuff that seemed to balance each other out, and I thought he was ok with it. Obviously I was wrong. Now I'm supposed to be doing all of it myself, when I'm three states away from everyone who loves us, and at the same time my job as a parent just got about ten times harder. I'm just so tired of feeling like a failure."

"What I'm hearing is a strong and capable person who has reached the end of her reserves," she summarized. "You are trying to take care of your kids and your parents, and everything at work and everything at home, and at the same time you are still trying to recover from the grief and trauma of losing your partner, and your son, and maybe your father, and trading in the life you knew for a new life that is still unfamiliar."

I nodded. She went on.

"And, as you mentioned, you're also struggling with very real and difficult changes in your body that go along with aging and perimenopause, all with no one to be there for you. It's really no wonder you're feeling sad and lonely."

Hearing the words "sad and lonely" applied to me—so simple and yet so precise—started the waterworks again. How could I not have seen it? In addition to complaining about me being a workaholic, Moose had often called me "Pollyanna," saying I never admitted that anything in my life wasn't perfect. I had always felt so lucky in life that it never seemed right to complain. But maybe, just maybe, I was now having some legitimate challenges that would benefit from being addressed head on.

"Why don't we plan to start there next week." This was a statement rather than a question, her skillful way of letting me know our time was up. "In the meantime, I'm going to suggest a little five-minute ritual for you to do every night before bed. Are you willing to do that?" I nodded. *I'm a good girl, I am.*

My assignment was to keep a notebook next to my bed and write down two things every night after a few minutes of slow breathing. First, I was supposed to write down a time in the day when I noticed one of my own unmet needs, and how it felt in my body when I noticed it. And second, write down a time that day when I noticed one of my needs being met, when I felt cared for, either by myself or by someone else.

When I got home that day, Kelsey met me dancing at the door.

"I'm a big sister!" She shoved her phone in my face. *OK, Jen, you've prepared for this.* I held her phone farther away so I could see the squishy red face wrapped in that ubiquitous pink and blue and white hospital blanket. Trans pride colors.

"Congratulations!" I hugged her. "What's her name?"

"Layla."

"That's pretty."

"Yeah."

"How's Amber doing?"

"Dad says she's fine. I didn't talk to her."

"And how's your dad?"

"He's good." She sounded a little tentative.

"Yeah?"

"Yeah, he looked so happy. Was he that happy when I was born?"

"Oh my gosh, absolutely he was! We were both thrilled when you arrived, you and Eliot." She smiled and went back to dancing and texting.

I went into my office and checked in with myself. *Now that it's happened, you can stop waiting for it.* Maybe it was because I'd already cried myself out earlier with Nancy, but I didn't feel that bad just then. I felt...neutral. Neither happy nor sad. Moose's new child was just a fact, not something that had to throw me into a tailspin. *Maybe I'm finally growing up after all.*

Over the next few weeks as I kept a journal, I began to notice all the things I was missing—my unmet needs. Some of these were fairly obvious: sleep, exercise, and (occasionally) sex. I craved healthy food but alternated between going hungry and stuffing myself with whatever junk food I could find. My unmet need for affection from my firstborn, accompanied by an ache in my chest, was a recurring theme. Other needs surprised me a little, like when I realized how much I craved affirmation at work, of the sort I used to get when I was everyone's favorite professor, beloved by my students, colleagues, and bosses alike.

But there were also times when I discovered my needs being met—when Kelsey gave me hugs for no reason; when Jamie sent funny texts, went running with my son, or brought over alcohol-free cocktails; when someone at work did their job extremely well and made my job easier, or thanked me for something.

At other times I met my own needs—taking walks and enjoying the hints of spring, preparing healthy lunches to eat at the office, or going to bed earlier. Nancy called this "parenting myself." I noticed that, when I did these things, they lifted some of the weight off my chest. A few times I even slept through the night.

After that first meeting, Nancy and I had virtual meetings one evening each week after work, and every time it seemed like I learned something new about myself. She always seemed to have a good question to ask that I hadn't thought of myself. It was like having a good mechanic. During one of our meetings Kelsey knocked and walked into my home office to tell me we were out of milk again. I sent her away till I was done.

"Who were you talking to?" she asked when I came out of the office. I hesitated for a moment, and then figured I might as well tell her.

"My therapist," I said.

"You have a therapist?" she asked, astonished.

"Yep."

"How come?" she asked. I laughed, but then realized she wasn't kidding. *Ah, the blissfulness of youth.*

"Ummm…" I decided she deserved the truth, even if not the whole truth. "This year has been full of big changes for me, for all of us. I'm stressed and I'm not sure I'm handling it very well, so I thought I could use a little help."

"Oh," she said, expressionless. Then, "How long will it last?"

I thought about it for a moment. "I don't know, actually. I've never done this before. I guess maybe till I feel better?" I shrugged. "We'll see."

"Oh," she said again. "Can we have pancakes for dinner?"

I laughed again. We should all bounce back so quickly. "Sure," I said. "But first we need milk."

I didn't feel like dealing with the hugeness of Meijer so I made a quick trip to the pharmacy, where I also picked up some psyllium husk. Nancy had suggested that adding fiber to my diet might help with the diarrhea. She had also urged me to find a different doctor, STAT.

When I got home from the store, Kelsey met me at the door and took the bags while I took my coat off. I went to the kitchen and started getting things out to make pancakes. She interrupted me with a big hug from behind.

"Poor Mom," she said. "I'm sorry you're stressed. You're doing a good job." That was a moment for my bedtime notebook. I turned around and hugged her back.

"Thank you, sweetie. That means a lot."

Chapter 23

A Doctor Who Knows from Menopause

Nancy had told me about something called the North American Menopause Society, which apparently had a website that listed practitioners nationwide who were certified in treating menopausal and perimenopausal patients. Unsurprisingly there weren't any in St. Jutta, so I picked a female MD about forty-five minutes away, Nikki Holiday, who was taking new patients. I explained my situation to a sympathetic-sounding woman with a strong Michigan accent (my name in her mouth sounded like "Junnifer"), who set me up with the first available appointment with "Dacktor Hal-iday."

When the day came, I had my calendar cleared of meetings and dropped my kids off at school so I could take the minivan. The Lansing Area Women's Health Clinic was on the second floor of a generic office park amid busy suburban sprawl. In the small waiting room were a middle-aged white woman and her adolescent daughter, filling out paperwork on a clipboard. I imagined they were there for the girl's first pelvic exam, or maybe to get her a prescription for the pill. A bored-looking pregnant woman with flaming pink hair sat scrolling on her phone.

I checked in at the receptionist's window, and as I turned to sit down with my own clipboard, I locked eyes with a Black person who I suspected was trans. We both smiled with our eyes and offered *sotto voce* hellos through our masks. I wondered how they felt about being at a "women's" health clinic, but supposed it was probably preferable to a waiting room full of cis men. I thought of Jamie and felt guilty again about my humiliating outburst. *Move on, Jen.*

When it was my turn, a woman too young for menopause called me back, measured and weighed me without comment, took my blood pressure, and led me into an examination room where she followed up on the health questionnaire I had filled out. I started feeling anxious about getting yelled at again, and by the time the doctor came in I had girded up my proverbial loins for more humiliation.

But when she entered, her vibe cleared up my mood almost immediately. She shook my hand and introduced herself as Nikki, and right away I liked her better than the last one. She looked a little bit older than I, maybe sixty or so, with friendly wrinkles around her soft, pale face. Her short hair was dyed brown, with a few gray roots showing. She was neither fat nor thin, neither tall nor short. Basically, an unremarkable, invisible middle-aged white lady. *Just like me.* I suddenly understood the incalculable value of diversity in medicine and felt bad that it took me so long to get it.

"So, you're going through 'the change,' eh?" she asked with a conspiratorial smile. "My condolences."

"Thanks," I laughed.

"I've been there and it's no fun at all. Tell me about your experience."

I told her everything, starting with the easier things—sweating, not being able to sleep, peeing myself, joint pain, forgetfulness. Eventually I worked my way up to the more embarrassing things—crying all the time, having uncharacteristic verbal outbursts, and gaining roughly ten pounds a year. (At least I didn't have to tell her about diarrhea. Nancy's recommendation about fiber was already helping.) After completing the litany I concluded, "And when I recently asked my last doctor about hormone replacement therapy, she cut me off and wouldn't even talk to me about it, as if I was asking for opioids or something."

"Was she younger?"

"Yeah."

"She probably went through med school in the early 2000s, when people were really freaking out about hormone therapy. They didn't get good education about menopause. The advice to women at the time was basically kind of just 'suck it up,' and unfortunately most medicine hasn't caught up with newer developments."

"Huh."

"Anyway, there are a few things we can talk about," she said. "First of all, I prefer the term 'menopausal hormone therapy' to 'hormone replacement therapy,' because 're-placement' implies there's something wrong with you. We're not replacing something your body *should* be making; you don't need to be *cured* from menopause. We're just trying to treat your symptoms, and hormones might or might not be a good option for doing that."

As a literary critic, I appreciated that reframing. I wondered if she'd had a liberal arts education.

"Secondly," she went on, "the fear about hormone therapy and breast cancer is largely an unfortunate misunderstanding created by media people who don't know how medical studies work. And women have been suffering needlessly for decades because of it. The facts are that for women in their early fifties, with no history of breast cancer, the long-term benefits of MHT can be tremendous, especially for the prevention of heart disease and osteoporosis, and maybe even colon cancer. And in the short term it can help with mood swings, weight gain, and sleep loss due to vasomotor symptoms."

"Vasomotor?"

"Hot flashes. Power surges, night sweats, whatever name you prefer for when your body heats up out of nowhere." I nodded, wondering if she had detected the tissues stuffed under my bra. "They're among the most common symptoms of perimenopause. Basically your hypothalamus overreacts to heat stimuli while it's getting used to there being less estrogen in your system."

"What joy."

"Isn't it? Weight gain and depression or mood swings are also extremely common with perimenopause, so it sounds like you're right on schedule. How's your libido?"

I told her I had two kids and a new job and sex was usually the last thing on my mind, but it didn't matter much because I was also currently single.

"OK, well just FYI, loss of libido is also pretty typical, as is pain during sex, so if that ever becomes an issue we can talk about it later. Some of the other symptoms you mentioned—joint pain, bladder control issues, and so forth—can sometimes be related to menopause but sometimes have other causes that just go along with normal aging."

"What about falling down?" I interrupted. "I seem to fall all the time now."

"It's not uncommon for older women to fall more often," she said. "It goes along with reduced muscle mass. I can recommend some core exercises if you'd like."

Fuck me, if one more person tells me to exercise...

"But let me just say," she said firmly, putting her hand on my arm, "in case you've been led to believe otherwise, *you haven't done anything wrong* and there is probably nothing wrong with you. Getting older is not a character flaw—it's actually a privilege. All of this is perfectly healthy and normal, even though it's disturbing and scary and feels really awful sometimes."

"But I should have been exercising all this time."

"Even people who exercise get diseases and disabilities," she said. "There's no right way to get older, and we all start out with different packages of genes and habits, so there's nothing to blame yourself for."

I thought about how much hatred I had directed at my body in recent months and suddenly felt great sadness and sympathy for it. *Poor body, you've been working so hard to keep going, even when your brain is constantly attacking you for doing precisely what you were designed to do. I'm sorry I've been so mean to you.*

She interrupted my thoughts. "So when was your last period?"

"Last May."

"Right. So medically we'd say you're perimenopausal, rather than post-menopausal, until you've gone a full year without a period. The good news is, you don't *have* to put up with these negative symptoms right now if you don't want to. Menopausal hormone therapy would likely bring you great relief, probably pretty quickly, especially from hot flashes and moodiness, which should also help you sleep. And based on your age and health history, the risks of negative side-effects is pretty low. You're kind of in the sweet spot. I'll give you some literature to take home so you can read about it."

That pleased me, as reading assignments always did, even though I already had a bunch of mostly unread books about it on my bedside table.

"If you decide you'd like to try MHT, I would recommend starting with an estradiol patch. You can try it for a few months and then we'll go from there."

"Can I start right now?" I didn't want to wait one more minute. She laughed.

"Yes, if you're sure, I can call in the prescription today." I assured her that I was. I left her office feeling grateful and hopeful, heard and seen.

In the car I listened to a podcast I had downloaded about menopause. The episode was on the impact of systemic racism in midlife women's health. However bad I had it, Black women predictably had it much worse because of health care disparities and racist policies and health care professionals—just like Melissa had told us back in January. Black women had disproportionately earlier menopause and more hysterectomies, which raised their risk of heart disease, but they also got disproportionately less hormone therapy than white women. Doctors apparently took Black women's suffering even less seriously than white women's, and researchers almost never bothered to study Black women in particular. I made a mental note to talk with the nursing and natural science department chairs about how we were addressing racial justice in our health curriculum.

I stopped at Meijer before going home, mostly to pick up my prescription but also to get the horrors of grocery shopping over with. I got a huge cart and bought doubles of everything in hopes of staving off my next grocery run. For dinner I picked up a bagged salad and a rotisserie chicken for me and Kelsey. Eliot would have to make do with frozen veggie burgers. Before the check-out lanes, saw a beautiful bouquet of tiny pink and white roses and got an idea.

"Are you free for dinner tonight question mark," I spoke into my phone. "Nothing fancy comma just chicken and salad period." The phone got all the spelling right on the first try. I texted the message to Jamie. We hadn't really seen each other since I visited her to ask for forgiveness a couple of weeks ago. I picked up the bouquet, and while I was still waiting for an actual human to check me out and bag my groceries, she texted back.

<Yes! What time?> A surge of joy went through my chest. We agreed she would come over after the bookstore closed at six.

"Hellooo!" I called out when I got home. "Can I get some help with groceries?" Kelsey came bounding down the stairs and I asked her to get her brother. By the time he came down Kelsey and I were mostly done bringing bags in.

"Jesus, look at all those plastic bags," he said.

"Thanks for buying my food, Mom," I said in a sing-song voice. "You're welcome, son!"

"Thank you," he said begrudgingly, "but couldn't you get reusable bags?"

"You're right," I said. Because he was. "But I need these for cat litter." He didn't respond but carried the last three bags into the kitchen.

"Who are these flowers for?" Kelsey asked.

"They're for Jamie. She's coming over for dinner," I said.

"Yay!" Kelsey said.

"Why?" Eliot asked.

"Just because."

"Yay!" Kelsey said again.

Eliot remarked, "You're in a good mood."

"Yes I am," I confirmed. "I had a good day." When I started telling them about my doctor's appointment Eliot rolled his eyes and went back upstairs, but Kelsey was rapt and had a dozen questions. I felt proud of myself for being a mother who talked to her daughter about menopause. I hoped it would serve her well someday. I wondered if I would live long enough to see her go through it.

After putting groceries away I went upstairs into the bathroom and closed the door. I opened the box of estradiol patches and took one out. It looked kind of like a band-aid. The doctor had told me to stick it to my lower abdomen. I did so anxiously—both excited that it might help and nervous that it might not. Then I did a couple of hours of work till Jamie came over, with mocktails for four ready to go in a frosty shaker. As she poured them into tiny antique tumblers, she remarked on the beautiful flowers. I told her they were for her. She handed me a drink and we looked at each other for a few seconds, eyes locked, both smiling stupidly.

"Can we eat? I'm starving!" said Kelsey.

"Seriously," Eliot added.

"Now now, my adolescent friends, your mother and I are having a moment," Jamie responded. Handing them their mocktails she said, "Here you go. Cheers. Shut up and drink while we finish."

She came to me and we embraced. When we parted, she picked up her mocktail and gave one to me.

"To your health," she said.

"And to yours," I responded. "And speaking of health..." Eliot groaned. "... I have so much to tell you!"

Before our April cabinet meeting, I had vowed to myself to get *one* good thing done for the faculty this year. The faculty had already signed their new contracts for the coming year because I hadn't managed to get approval for targeted raises in time, but I was determined to fix the inequities before the next academic year. Better late than never, I hoped.

The week before, the VP for advancement and I had talked to the erstwhile Greta Thunberg Climate and Environmental Justice chair donor for two hours over Zoom (she was at her home in Sedona, with giant red rocks visible through the window behind her). We had convinced her to let go of the title that so offended a few of the board members. Instead, she agreed it could be innocuously named the Chair of Environmental Studies, which was already an improvement for the institution, since there was currently an interdisciplinary minor but no actual department or even a director of environmental studies. The position would be for a tenured, senior professor—someone who couldn't easily be pushed around—with expertise in ecological science or environmental ethics and policy. The job would be specifically oriented toward putting climate and environmental issues on the front burner of the school, and would come with a course release and a generous departmental budget so the person could bring in big-name speakers and coordinate programs with other faculty. She seemed content with what we had worked out, and I felt proud of myself for helping to garner such a large gift for the academic sector.

My boss was happy, too—happy enough that I wanted to strike while the iron was hot on the salary question, before things went back to normal.

"It's time," I said, when the agenda came to me. "We can't wait another year to create salary equity among the mid-career faculty. Sam, would you do the honors?"

I had worked with the CFO to create some tables to illustrate the problem. It wasn't easy, since the faculty was so small that it was difficult to put up data without everyone knowing exactly whose salary was whose. We ultimately consolidated the faculty into large blocks—male and female, in three ranks. We also combined departments into two divisions – arts, humanities, and social sciences as one category, natural sciences, health sciences, and business as the other. (The "useless" majors and the useful ones, as popularly beheld.)

Our first slide compared the useless and useful majors by rank. It was painfully obvious that the faculty in the useless departments were significantly underpaid compared to their counterparts in the useful majors, and the gap got bigger as faculty got older.

"That's just supply and demand," said the COO. You can't expect to pay a PhD economist the same thing as an English professor."

"I agree, to an extent," I said. "It's true that—at hiring time—there are many more candidates for arts and humanities jobs than for business or nursing. But the marketability of those folks also wanes over time. Someone who's been teaching management to undergraduates for the past 20 years is simply not going to just walk out the door and get hired by a corporation for six figures."

The COO shifted in his chair.

"And meanwhile," I kept my voice calm, "over time, the arts and humanities faculty do far more than their share of the work of this institution, including teaching core classes for huge numbers of science and business majors. We cannot simply keep exploiting them because we think they have no other options. That is antithetical to a liberal arts ethos, in my opinion."

The next slide broke down male and female faculty by rank. There was only a small gender discrepancy among newer faculty, thanks mainly to nursing, but between the male and female associate and full professors, the gap was pronounced. Some people actually gasped when they saw it. I explained anyway.

"A female professor hired in the 1990s earns about ten percent less than a male professor hired in the 90s with the same degree. This adds up to hundreds of thousands of dollars over a career, which is especially problematic at retirement time. That is simply unacceptable. We all know how much weight the mid-career female faculty are pulling with regard to academic service, advising, and committee assignments. Sam?"

The CFO pulled up the next slide and I went on.

"As it happens, we are also spending tens of thousands of dollars each year on part-time, adjunct faculty to teach one or two classes here and there. Many of these instructors do not have PhDs, or even degrees in the specialties they are teaching."

I couldn't offer any examples without calling out specific individuals, so I left it at that.

"Meanwhile, a high number of specialized classes taught by full-time faculty are under-enrolled. My proposal, therefore..." I nodded at Sam, who moved to the next slide, "is to work with the faculty to update their programs in ways that can be sustained solely by the full-time faculty in those programs, without the need for part-time help except to cover sabbaticals. With the money we save on adjunct instructors, we can afford to bump up the salaries of those who have dedicated their lives to this institution and been grossly underpaid for decades."

I waited a moment for this to sink in before heading into my conclusion. The COO looked like he wanted to disagree, but he waited impatiently for me to finish.

"In addition, I have discovered large pots of unused, un-designated funds sitting in various pockets throughout the academic budget."

Sam put up another slide, listing budget lines and small endowments in various departments that had $5,000 here, $8,000 there, for projects that people had entirely forgotten about.

"These add up to about $75,000, which can also help offset the salary bumps. It won't make up for all the years of lost earnings, but it will help a little in the final years of their careers, and it will get St. Margaret's on the right track going forward. Basic fairness is *literally* the least we can offer to people who spend their lives working for our students."

I nodded at Sam. He turned the slides off while I turned the room lights back on and sat down. I was sweating, but in what felt like a normal way for someone giving a speech about something important, rather than a hot flash kind of way.

"Yes, thank you, Jennifer," Norm said. "In the coming weeks and months we'll be working together on a plan to get salary bumps in place as soon as possible."

"Thanks, Norm. I'm planning to get it done by the end of this fiscal year," I interjected with a smile. "Sam and I have already worked it out. I'll come see you about it ASAP."

"Yes, we'll see how things develop. Athletics is our next agenda item..."

Chapter 24

Mothers' and Non-Mothers' Days

In early May, someone leaked a draft of a majority Supreme Court opinion on a Mississippi abortion law. It was shocking—though no real surprise—that SCOTUS's new majority was planning to vote to overturn Roe v. Wade. A bunch of red states had already created "trigger laws" that would eliminate rights immediately upon the court's official decision. All that was left was to await the blessed day when Christian theocracy would be restored in America, just like the Puritans intended. (Except even Puritans didn't care about fetuses before quickening—but whatever. *History schmistory.*)

Michigan's abortion laws were currently ambiguous. Technically abortion had been outlawed in 1931. Without Roe to stop them, conservative prosecutors could potentially start enforcing a ban whenever the SCOTUS decision was official. The governor, "that woman from Michigan," and Planned Parenthood had already filed lawsuits to try to protect abortion rights in the state. And the attorney general, also a woman (and an out lesbian), had signaled her refusal to enforce the 1931 law. But the majority conservative state legislature made it unclear what options would be open to pregnant people in the coming months.

An impromptu "Bans Off Our Bodies" protest rally was planned for the next evening on the capitol lawn in Lansing. Jamie was planning to go and invited me along. I thought about my kids and their almost-adult bodies—Kelsey still getting used to having her period, Eliot still too awkward to talk about condoms. And of course I had no idea what Anna thought about contraception. As much as I wanted to be a grandmother someday, I didn't want that day to be too soon. (Plus, having experienced the messiness of miscarriage, I knew how close it came to what many people thought of as abortion, and I didn't want anyone to have to fight for the right to life-saving or fertility-saving health care.)

So I invited my kids to the rally. Kelsey enthusiastically agreed, which I had expected, but I was shocked when Eliot said he and Anna wanted to go too. Apparently Anna was currently taking AP Government at the high school, and the teacher (god bless her) had gotten the students stirred up about SCOTUS suddenly going back on fifty years of legal precedent and women's bodily autonomy.

Saturday afternoon, the five of us piled into Jamie's Subaru and drove to Michigan's capital city. The car ride soundtrack was provided by a Swedish singer named Robyn that the kids knew but I didn't. We stopped on our way for doughnuts at the Mennonite bakery, its shop full of hand-made Americana tchotchkes, fragrant barrels of last fall's apples, and random gifts like puzzles and windchimes. A short young woman in a dowdy homemade dress and apron, with a lace covering over her tight hair bun, took our order, filled up our bag with cinnamon-sugar-covered treasures, and sent us on our merry way. I wondered what she would think if she knew where we were going. I knew some Mennonites who were for abortion rights, but I suspected these might not be those kinds of Mennonites.

It was drizzling when we arrived downtown. We found a spot in a parking garage and walked a couple of blocks to the capitol—a building of neo-classical design, symmetrical and imposing, made of light-colored stone, not too tall except for the elongated white dome on top. I felt a strange surge of pride in my new home state, followed by a twinge of guilt that I had never once taken my kids to Trenton, even for the Women's March in 2017. *How are you over 50 and this is your first protest rally?* I had obviously been way too comfortable till now. Maybe all this upheaval in my life was slowly making me more sensitive to other people's suffering.

A few hundred people in raincoats, punctuated by colorful umbrellas and signs, gathered in the center of the lawn at the bottom of the steps. A handmade sign with a uterus said DON'T TREAD ON ME. Several people wore hot pink Planned Parenthood scarves and carried hot pink signs that said PROTECT SAFE, LEGAL ABORTION. Another group carried shiny, mass-produced posters with black fists that read REPRODUCTIVE RIGHTS ARE HUMAN RIGHTS.

The program was provided by a handful of Democrats from the state legislature, who spoke about how bad it would be for pregnant people—especially poor people and people of color—if the 1931 law went back into effect in Michigan. Meanwhile, activists were working the crowd, circulating petitions to get a reproductive freedom amendment for the state Constitution on the November 2022 ballot. Those of us over 18—Jamie, Anna, and I—all signed. Jamie also signed up to collect signatures in St. Jutta before the July 1 deadline. I wasn't sure what my boss would think of me doing that, so I promised Jamie I would send folks to the bookshop if they wanted to sign. Anna planned to bring in her over-18 friends, too.

We were hungry after the rally and Jamie took us to a Korean restaurant she knew near the Amtrak station.

"I've never had Korean food," Kelsey said. No one else had either. I didn't say out loud that I'd been prejudiced against it ever since smelling kimchee for the first time in my dorm at Madison.

"You're going to love it, trust me," said Jamie. "Or at least you'll love some of it."

Apparently the usual thing was to cook meat on a little grill in the middle of the table, but out of respect for Eliot she ordered a vegetarian spread for us all—big bowls of soup, giant pancakes covered in scallions that we cut into slices with scissors, crispy tofu, chewy noodles that reminded me of gnocchi, and tiny bowls containing about ten different kinds of kimchee of varying spiciness. I tried everything and Jamie was right—it was all tasty, and some of it was positively delicious. There were little red bean buns for dessert.

"I first started eating Korean food when I lived in Chicago," Jamie told us. "It was a revelation." She closed her eyes, summoning the memory. "One of my favorite places did Mexican-Korean fusion and put kimchee on tacos. Mmmm!"

"I've been to Chicago for conferences a couple of times," I said, "but I've never really managed to explore the city." I couldn't believe how lame that sounded.

"Let me know next time you go and I'll give you some recommendations." Then she added with a smile, "Or better yet, take me with you! I'll show you all the best places."

"I wanna go too!" said Kelsey.

"Yeah, me too," said Anna with a smile. She looked at Eliot, who briefly looked like a deer in headlights before silently eating another chewy noodle-thingy with his disposable chopsticks. I was happy his girlfriend seemed to be having fun and hoped maybe it would give me a tiny bit more cred with my son.

"So Anna, are you excited about nursing school?" I asked.

"So excited," she beamed. "I'm rooming with my friend Hannah. She's also doing the BSN."

"How far away is EMU?" Kelsey asked, reaching for some more kimchee.

"It's like, an hour and a half," Anna said. Kelsey looked at Eliot with concern.

"What?" he asked, eyes wide.

We all laughed, and even Eliot smirked, but I felt a pang in my chest. There was no telling what the future held for him and Anna, but chances were pretty good that a break-up was in their future. I already felt sorry for both of them, especially whoever got dumped. *Heartbreak is a quintessential life experience, Jen. They'll figure it out.*

Our good mood continued on the ride home. Despite the news and the weather, I think we felt happy that we had done something, in a crowd of people who were also doing something, and who cared about things we cared about. I felt hopeful that maybe Michigan could be a safe place for my kids to grow into adulthood, and I felt a renewed sense of purpose about helping to educate the next generation of Michigan adults. I made a mental note to work with college staff and faculty this summer to get out the vote in November.

Then I remembered something Nancy said, when I had complained to her about how my mental notes didn't work anymore. She had suggested that, rather than berate myself for forgetting things, I could find some gentle ways to accept and accommodate my changing brain. I could try a different strategy. So I got out my phone and sent myself a quick email reminder. That way I could forget all about it for now, and it would be waiting in my in-box later when I could sit down and think, send a proper email, or put a meeting on my calendar. After pressing "send," I smiled and rested my head back on the car seat.

"What is it?" Jamie looked at me, briefly taking her eyes off the road.

"Nothing."

"You look happy."

"I feel happy." It didn't seem right, given the horrible state of the world, but it was true.

"Yaaaay, Mom's happy!" Kelsey said, rubbing my shoulders from the back seat, like I was a boxer in the ring.

On Mother's Day, Fiona woke me up by playing with the glass of water on my bedside table. I looked at my phone to check the time. Six forty-five. I had slept through the night. I wanted to roll over and go back to sleep, and I tried for a few minutes, but my bladder insisted upon itself. Around seven I got up and limped to the bathroom on my sore feet, which always needed a little extra time to wake up and face the day. When I came out of the bathroom, Kelsey was standing in the hall with a steaming cup of coffee.

"Happy Mother's Day!" she said, giving me a hug with her free arm, extending the coffee cup arm far away from us without spilling.

"Oh, thank you sweetie." I squeezed her and kissed her head. "How did you remember?"

"Of course I remembered," she said. "But Dad also texted yesterday to remind us."

That was a surprise, but a welcome one. I had lucked into marrying a man whose mother had trained him to shower her with love and attention at designated times, so birthdays and Mother's Days had always been nice events for me. Moose always made the kids get up and cook breakfast, and usually we all went for a walk or a movie or something, and then we'd go visit the grandmas in the afternoon and evening.

"Go back to bed and have your coffee!" she ordered. I did as I was told.

"Thank you, darling," I said, in my best imitation of Jamie.

"What do you want for breakfast?" she asked. "Jamie's coming over with mimosas."

When she went back downstairs, Fiona followed her and I was alone with my thoughts, which were a little dark. This year was my first Mother's Day as a single mom, as well as being far away from my own mother figures. Since I had the time, I did what Nancy said and checked in with my body to see how I felt physically. I noticed a heavy place on my chest, fogginess in my head, and some tension in my face right under my eyes. I took some deep breaths and told myself it was ok to feel sad. At the same time, I reminded myself that feelings are temporary and tried to let the tension go.

After a couple of minutes the worst of it had passed. Fiona came back in and stomped on my chest where the heavy place used to be, and head butted my nose, and it was cute. I decided to call my own mom before I got too distracted.

"Hi, Ma, happy Mother's Day!"

"Oh, thank you, honey! Happy Mother's Day to you, too."

"What are you all up to today?"

"Oh, nothing special. Your father and I might go see a matinee with your aunt and uncle, since you're not here." As an adult, I had often included my aunt and uncle in Mother's and Father's Day celebrations, because they, too, had been a major part of my support system growing up. As an only child, I had been showered with adults' attention my entire life.

I ignored my mother's subtle guilt trip and said, "That sounds fun. I'm sorry I'm not there to take you all out, but I'm glad you're still getting together."

"Well what are you doing today?" I told her how my day had started so auspiciously. We talked for a few more minutes and worked out a few details for their upcoming graduation visit to Michigan. Then, just as I began to smell bacon, I also heard the smoke alarm going off and the kids yelling at each other. *Just turn down the heat, kiddos.* I told my mom I loved her and headed downstairs to rescue the kids.

In the kitchen, Eliot was mixing up pancake batter and Kelsey was wrestling with some extra-curly bacon in the cast iron pan. I put my arm around her as I turned the burner down from high to low, then I opened the back door and grabbed a dish towel to wave under the smoke detector. The kitchen smelled like coffee and charred flesh, with just a hint of Eliot's manly hair products.

When the beeping finally stopped, I closed the door. Kelsey directed me to sit down at the table, where there was an envelope waiting that said "MOM" with hearts all around it. I recognized the card from the rack in Jamie's bookstore. Both kids had signed it, which made me feel warm in the places where the tension had been a few minutes ago. My ridiculously adorable daughter poured my second cup of coffee.

When Jamie arrived, everyone sat down and we all ate our pancakes and drank our alcohol-free mimosas, and everyone except Eliot had bacon. Then the kids cleaned up the kitchen while Jamie and I lounged on the sofa and made plans for the rest of the day.

The weather was chilly but sunny, so we hit the bike path. We dusted off our bikes, which had been sitting sadly in the garage all winter, and pumped up their tires. The path was only a few blocks away and was mercifully flat, traveling along a former train track. My unused quads were burning within minutes, but it felt good to be moving my body and flying through the countryside. Every now and then we passed people walking their dogs or pushing strollers. Occasionally a serious cyclist overtook us and left us in their dust. The trail was dotted with patches of white birch trees, whose leaves flickered delicately above our heads. Kelsey squealed and swerved to avoid running over a tiny snake.

Eliot turned around after a couple of miles, having done his filial duty, but the rest of us kept going at Jamie's urging. About four miles out of town, we arrived at a lonely little cemetery at a rural crossroads. Some kind of grain elevator and a broken-down barn stood across from it, with an abandoned stone house on the opposite corner. We wandered among the gravestones and flowering trees for a while, sipping from our water bottles. We finally lay down on the grass in a patch of sun, next to an ancient oak tree, between MARY DYKSTRA, BELOVED WIFE AND MOTHER and MULDER (no further information).

"I wonder what Mary died of," Kelsey said pensively.

"Would you rather die suddenly or slowly?" Jamie asked.

"Ugh, neither," Kelsey answered. "I want to live forever." *Just wait till you're my age and you're so tired death starts to sound like a relief.*

"I guess I haven't thought about it that carefully," I said, "but I suppose I need time to say goodbye to everyone and clean up my messes before I go."

Jamie smiled warmly. "Because of course you would be thinking of everyone else first."

Kelsey threw her arms around me. "You can't die, Mom!"

I hugged her back. "I can and I will, but hopefully not too soon. What about you, Jamie?"

"I kind of hope for a sudden death," she said looking up at the sky. "Like, dropping dead of a heart attack while running on a gorgeous day like this, or crashing into the ocean on my way home from some epic vacation in New Zealand, never to be seen again." She laughed heartily when Kelsey and I both cried out in dismay.

The whole conversation reminded me that I needed to update my last will and testament, now that I didn't have a husband anymore. A few months ago that thought would have filled me with sadness and dread, but at that moment it just seemed like a practical matter that I could take care of as soon the academic year ended. I already had a lawyer.

After an hour of cloud watching and conversation on Jamie's blanket, we rode back home at a leisurely pace and said our goodbyes. The Mother's Day I had been dreading had turned out nearly perfect after all.

After I'd already gotten into bed that night and was working on emails, my phone rang. It was Moose. I answered tentatively.

"Happy Mother's Day."

"Thanks?" It came out as a question, sounding ruder than I meant it. "Thanks for reminding the kids."

"Sure thing. You deserve it." I didn't know what to say to that. What anyone deserved or didn't deserve was becoming less and less clear to me. I changed the subject.

"How's everything in Costa Rica?"

"Yeah, fine," he said tentatively. "I'm, uh, thinking about flying up there for Eliot's graduation, if that's OK with you."

I sighed inwardly. He should have talked to me about this months ago. Then again, I was a bit difficult to talk to months ago.

"Of course," I managed. "He'd be devastated if you didn't come."

"Great. Do you, uh, have any room for us to stay with you?"

Dude, are you fucking kidding me? I took a deep breath. "My parents are staying with us, but I'll see if there's room in the college guest house that weekend." Silence. "It's just a couple of blocks away."

"Oh, ok. Thanks."

"Yup. Do your parents want to come?"

"Yes, if that's ok."

"Of course it's ok," I said, trying not to sound like a nag. "I'll reserve a room for them too. But I'd appreciate it if you could handle all the transportation to and from the airport for you and your folks. We have a lot going on and only the one car."

"Sure, of course," he said. "I'll rent a car."

I promised to email him all the information he needed, and then I waited to see if there was anything else. Nothing came. "Well, thanks for calling."

When we hung up, I did another body scan. I realized I had been waiting for that particular shoe to drop and it was a bit of a relief that it finally had. My shoulders had parked themselves up near my ears, so I deliberately shifted them down and wiggled them a bit. My chest was tight, so I took some deep breaths. For once I didn't feel like crying. Instead, I felt a small hint of pride for having conducted myself like a grown-up.

Nay, like a low-key goddess.

I sent myself an email to make reservations at the guest house first thing in the morning, and slept that night like the dead.

Chapter 25

Commencements

Eliot's graduation weekend approached, and the day before was a ridiculous whirlwind of comings and goings. I picked up my parents and got them installed in our guest room-slash-office. Moose got himself and his parents from the airport to the guest house on the campus of the College of St. Margaret, in beautiful St. Jutta, Michigan. I had forgotten he'd been there once before, when he came for some last-minute house-hunting without us. That seemed like years ago.

We all gathered for dinner at our house. I didn't cook, but I had gotten a bunch of prepared foods and arranged them buffet-style on the kitchen island. I had ordered my mother to be pleasant to Moose for the kids' and my sake, and thankfully she was on her best behavior. Kelsey helped a lot by keeping the grandmothers entertained with tales of middle school drama.

My dad and Moose's dad had always gotten along, even if they weren't exactly friends. They had a friendly, decades-long, Mets-versus-Phillies rivalry, united in their hatred of the Yankees after Steinbrenner fired Yogi Berra. Eliot sat close to his grandfathers, listening without comment. Apart from running, sports had never been his thing.

Moose and I floated from conversation to conversation, avoiding finding ourselves in the same one at the same time. After dinner I had to fight my mother-in-law for the right to clean up the kitchen, but with Moose's help I prevailed. We called it an early night and he took his folks back to the guest house. The kids and my dad went off to their rooms and my mom hung around for a cup of tea.

"How are *you* doing, Jennifer?" she asked as the kettle heated up. "This all must be so hard on you."

"I think I'm ok, Mom," I said truthfully. "It's all a bit weird but it's ok. I'm happy for Eliot to be properly celebrated by his family."

"It was nice to see Howard and Marie again," she admitted, "and I'm glad at least Moose showed up for his son."

I ignored the tone of the latter part of her sentence and focused on the first. "Yes, it was really great that they came." *OMG, you sound like Norm.* "That all of you came. I know it means a lot to Eliot, even if he doesn't know how to express it." I hastened to add, "It means a lot to me, too."

She clucked her tongue and made a sympathetic face. "Oh, my poor girl." She gave me a hug. Her body felt small and frail, as if I could crush her. "You're such a good girl."

"Thanks, Mom."

"We're so proud of you."

"Thanks." I felt awkward, but also lucky to be from a family that mostly said nice things to each other, apart from the occasional fat-shaming. She squeezed me one last time and took her tea off to bed.

I had been sleeping somewhat better lately, but after all the stimulation that night I couldn't turn my brain off. I ended up turning on the light and answering emails till almost 2:00 a.m. Then I slept a few hours till it was time to make the coffee before my guests awoke.

While I was puttering in the kitchen, Eliot entered in his cap and gown. My chest seized and my eyes welled up, but I didn't immediately start bawling, so maybe the MHT was starting to work. I threw my arms around him and squeezed hard, eliciting an "Ugh" under his breath, and then finally an "Ok" and a begrudging hug in return. I let go before my nose started oozing onto his cheap-blue-polyester-covered shoulders. I noted with pride that he had ironed the gown without melting it, per my instructions.

"You look great, hon." I grabbed a tissue and tried to act normal. "When will you be home?"

The St. Jutta public schools had a special graduation day tradition. First they held commencement rehearsal in the morning, and then they packed all the seniors onto buses and took them on a memory lane tour—first to the elementary school, then the middle school, then back to the high school. At each school they walked the halls while teachers, students, and staff stood by and cheered.

"The usual time," he said. We'd figure out all the evening logistics later. I planned to work a half day at the office, leaving my parents and Moose and his folks to their own devices while the kids and I were out. I felt a bit guilty about this, so I kept chanting to myself: *They are grown-ass adults.*

As it turned out, the adults were fine. My dad rested at home and my mom took a long walk with her ankle weights on. Moose and his folks discovered Meijer to their great delight, especially the rows and rows of all kinds of booze on offer, right there in the grocery store. Ah, the everyday delights of middle America.

Marie made a huge pot of *penne* for dinner, complete with her mother's classic *sugo*, along with a big platter of sautéed spinach and some crusty garlic bread. Whoever sat near us in the gym was going to get a nose full, but it was delicious. Moose had picked out some bottles of chianti and poured some for everyone, even tiny amounts for the kids.

"To the graduate," he toasted, raising a glass. "We're proud of you, son." We all answered in kind and drank. Eliot looked embarrassed. Kelsey made a sour face.

I had forgotten how fun and festive it was to have a house full of loud family. A mix of gratitude and nostalgia swelled through me. They weren't technically all my family anymore, but they were still my kids' family, and just then it seemed close enough. I wished Jamie was there to see it. I texted her and reminded her to come over later for cake and a drink after the shop closed.

With much chaos, we all made it to the high school in time for Eliot to line up and us to find bleachers close to the ground, so the grandparents didn't have to climb too far. Unbelievably, I made it through "Pomp and Circumstance" and the whole ceremony without crying. *Thanks, hormone patch.* Except for Anna and a few kids from the cross country team, I didn't recognize many of the one hundred or so graduates, but I clapped for every single one. I limited myself to a short "whoop" when my firstborn's name was called, and it was easily drowned out by his father's unabashed cheering.

I missed seeing all the kids we'd known for years, who would soon be graduating without us in New Jersey, whose futures would remain mostly unknown apart from an occasional Facebook update. *Life goes on, Jen.* After the ceremony we all milled about on the school lawn. Kids posed with each other while older folks took photos, the last bits of evidence of our offspring's childhoods.

The grandparents looked like wilting plants so most of us left. Anna would bring Eliot back to the house later. At home Moose poured more wine. Jamie came over and entertained everyone in the living room while I put the vegan icing on the vegan cake that Kelsey and I had made earlier from a box. When Eliot and Anna arrived, a loud cheer went up. Introductions and more hugs ensued. Cake was cut, wine was drunk, stories were told. It felt like a proper party.

When I started picking up cake plates to take to the kitchen, Anna jumped up and helped.

"Hey, thanks!" I said, wiping powdered sugar off the counters with a sponge. "How do you feel?"

"Good," she said, shrugging.

"How was the walk through all your old schools today?"

"It was really fun," she said. "I got to see some of my old teachers." She took out her phone. "My kindergarten teacher gave me this." She showed me a picture of her own kindergarten photo, with a note of congratulations on the back.

"Aww, that's sweet," I said. "I don't think poor Eliot had ever even been inside those schools before." I was about to give into my usual guilt about uprooting him, but instead I decided to believe that our move was quite possibly one of the best things that had ever happened to him. I pivoted. "But I know he's very happy we came here this year."

She beamed. Whatever the future held, they were happy together for now.

A little while later, the big kids were supposed to head out to their "all-night party," designed to keep the seniors from drinking themselves into oblivion on their first night of freedom. (It didn't actually go all night. I guessed some committee had decided it would be sufficient to keep them busy into the wee hours, till they'd tired themselves out beyond the point of any serious mischief.) Eliot was having trouble extricating himself from his grandmothers so I intervened.

"Hey, hon," I put my hand on his shoulder, "I think Anna is about ready to go."

"Ok," he stood up.

"We're so proud of you, grandson," my dad said. His other grandparents concurred.

"Have fun," I said to them at the door. "Please be careful."

"We will," Eliot answered, with only mild irritation.

Moose's parents decided to take a "post-prandial walk" back to the guest house and my parents went off to bed. I went back into the kitchen to putter. After a few minutes Kelsey went upstairs to Facetime with her friends, and Moose and Jamie were left alone in the living room.

"Kelsey tells me you've really been there for them this year," I heard him say.

"I adore them," she said in return. "I can't imagine my life without them now!"

"Well, thanks."

"Don't mention it."

There was a moment of silence before he said, "I pretty much screwed them over last summer. All three of them." Jamie said nothing. I held my breath. Finally he added, "Luckily Jen's a fucking superhero."

"She absolutely is," Jamie said. "But that doesn't mean it's been easy on her. Or any of them."

"Yeah."

"Well I'm glad to meet you again under happy circumstances," she said after another pause. I heard them getting up and saying their goodbyes.

A moment later she was in the kitchen giving me a hug. "Thanks for the cake, darling." She held me away by the shoulders, her smiling eyes piercing into mine. "You're amazing," she whispered. My stomach fluttered. "Take care of yourself and text me when I can see you again."

"You know I will."

When she left, Moose came into the kitchen. I was wiping down the counters and didn't make eye contact. As cheerfully as I could I said, "Well, he did it."

"He did," Moose agreed. "So did you, Jen."

"Ha," I said. "Just barely."

"No, I mean it, Jen. You got him through this year basically on your own. I've been a total shit-head." *Damn straight you have.* I scrubbed the sink harder. "I don't know what I was thinking, leaving the way I did. I mean I don't..." he hesitated, "I guess I don't regret leaving. But I do regret the way I left. You deserved better."

I was overwhelmed with a flurry of thoughts and feelings—sadness, dissatisfaction, indignance, humiliation, rage, resignation, relief. But my feelings weren't really his business anymore. "It's done now, Moose," I said, still scrubbing. "I'll be fine, and you can still be here for your kids. They still need you."

"Actually, Amber and I are thinking of moving back to New Jersey soon."

"What?" I finally turned to him, sponge dripping on the floor. "No more *pura vida*?"

"Nah," he almost laughed. "It's great but it's too far away for real life. At least for now. She wants to be near her parents while Layla's growing up, and I know my folks want me back too."

"That's smart. I'm really glad our kids got to spend so much time with their grandparents growing up." My voice caught and my chest ached. I hoped my parents would make it to Kelsey's graduation. *Stop being so morbid, Jen.* "And it would be great if the kids could visit you and my parents at the same time."

"Yeah, it was good to see them," he said. "I can check in on them too, now and then. Are they OK?" I filled him in on my dad's various ailments, and told him I was certain my mom had undiagnosed ADHD that had gotten so much worse since she'd gotten an iPhone. He laughed and said, sounding surprised, "I've actually kind of missed them."

"I'm sure they've missed you too." *Or they would have if they didn't feel the need to hate you on my behalf.* "Anyway," I said, drying my hands on a dish towel, "I've got to go now."

In order to avoid hanging out with Moose for too long, I had volunteered to help chaperon and clean up after the not-really-all-night party (against Eliot's wishes, of course). My leaving would also give Moose some time alone with Kelsey, who I thought deserved a little individual attention. They planned to have a sing-along watch party of *Hamilton* together for old time's sake. It was their thing. Both of them knew all the words. I hoped my parents wouldn't mind too much. I had put a loud fan in their room in case they needed a noisemaker.

I went upstairs and stood in front of my closet, staring, wondering what to wear, anxious about being the oldest and fattest mother there. I took a deep breath and tried to channel Jamie. *Life's too short to give a fuck about how big your belly is.* I also remembered what Nancy said about gratitude. I said thank you to my body for getting me this far in relatively great health, for enabling me to be a mother, and for letting me have an interesting career and see cool things in the world.

I finally decided on basics, changing out of my dress into jeans and a St. Jutta Saints Cross Country t-shirt. Just for fun I added a chunky beaded choker that Kelsey had once picked out for me on a visit to Chinatown, that I loved but hadn't worn since becoming a provost. It looked kind of random but I thought Jamie would approve.

The high school had been decked out in red and gold balloons. There were inflatable games, laser tag, and a bunch of tables for blackjack and 21. The indoor pool was open for swimming, but I noticed there were no girls swimming—I guessed they had worked too hard on their hair to mess it up tonight. A booth with a fan in the floor blew dollar bills around and kids inside the booth had fifteen seconds to catch as many as possible. And in the kitchen there was a prize counter set up, where kids could trade in their tickets for rewards, like candy or gift cards.

I was assigned to the food area, a buffet overflowing with baked goods, sandwiches, individually-wrapped snacks, and cold drinks in plastic bottles that I knew would piss off Eliot. *Plastic is the devil.*

There were indeed some young, lithe mothers there who must have been barely out of high school themselves when their babies arrived. There were even a few flannel-clad dads helping out at the party. But as it turned out, the majority of volunteers were forty- and fifty-something women, many of them plump like me, just here to celebrate their children's achievements and be good citizens by supporting their local high school.

I relaxed into the moment. I recognized a couple of parents from cross country, met several new people, and enjoyed interacting with all the kids on the cusp of adulthood. Anna greeted me warmly, Eliot less warmly. After a few hours of games the kids were all gathered into the auditorium to watch a hypnotist make a dozen of their classmates do silly things on stage. Then grand prizes were announced, the kids dispersed, and the parents cleaned up. All in all, it seemed like a successful event.

I got home around 2:00 a.m. and left the porch light on for Eliot. I crept up the creaky stairs and found Kelsey half asleep in her bed, watching some video.

"Hey. How was *Hamilton*?"

"Good. Dad forgot a lot of the words."

"He's probably out of practice." She yawned. "Go to sleep, sweets." She rolled over and turned off the light without protest.

I brushed my teeth, put on my pajamas, and sank into bed. As I lay there, my mind wandered to my parents downstairs. I thought of Moose and his parents sleeping at the unfamiliar guest house. I thought of Eliot out with Anna somewhere, probably her house, hopefully safe. I realized I'd been holding my breath and tried to fill my lungs to the brim as I congratulated myself for making it through this day that I'd been dreading.

You are a fucking superhero, Jen. I'm really proud of you.

❋

By the time St. Margaret's commencement day came around, I was already sick of graduations, but also desperate for the academic year to end. The faculty were utterly burned out, after another year of dealing with students who were utterly burned out. I had done my best to support them over the past two semesters, but the stream of big and small dramas had been almost constant. Finals week had been even worse, bringing with it an onslaught of plagiarism cases, grade complaints, and end-of-year partying casualties.

We were all just done.

On my walk to work I scanned my phone for the day's headlines. The news was mostly terrible, as usual, but on the upside, Kate Bush was having a renaissance. Perhaps related to 80s nostalgia, there was also an article about how the nation was entering a "menopause gold rush" thanks to women my age. I couldn't help clicking on it.

I learned that apparently discussing menopause was "no longer taboo" because some Gen X celebrities were admitting they were no longer of child-bearing age. Middle-aged women have money to spend and bodies needing accommodation, the article said, hence the rush of new businesses. One "meno-preneur" was quoted as saying, "Every woman who goes through menopause says it's like she's the first person on earth who has ever done it because no one knows how to help."

I felt slightly vindicated. Then I tripped and almost fell. *One thing at a time, Jen. You can't afford a broken bone.*

When I crossed the street onto campus, there were graduates in robes and families scattered around on the lawns, hugging and taking photos. It felt festive, and I did my best to put my fatigue aside and get in a festive mood myself.

This is a big day for them, and they went through a lot to get here. The ceremony began at 2:00 p.m., so I picked up my robe from the office and went to line up with the administrators and faculty for our processional at 1:30.

"Hello, Jennifer," Vivan said. She was the faculty marshal, so she stood at the front of the faculty line carrying a large ceremonial mace. She looked dignified in her black robe and mortar board. "Are you ready for your debut as reader of the names?"

"I'll do my best," I said. "I've been practicing."

"I'm sure you'll be fine. It will be nice to have a woman doing it for a change. It's been a while." *No pressure.* "I wanted to thank you, by the way. For the raises."

"Oh, you're welcome. You've earned it."

"It means a lot to all of us. It's been a long time since we've felt appreciated by the administration."

"I do appreciate your work very much," I said genuinely. "It wasn't that long ago that I was faculty and I remember how demoralizing it can be. I'm sorry the raises can't be bigger but I'll keep working on it."

When the time came, Pomp and Circumstance started up again and we all processed into the gym, where it was normally held. In 2020 commencement had been canceled altogether, and in 2021 they had risked an outdoor ceremony. But May in Michigan is still a gamble, so for the class of 2022, the decision was made to gamble with Covid instead of the weather. Six seniors were already in quarantine after partying during exam week. (Thankfully it was not I but the VP of student affairs who'd had to inform their parents.)

As provost I was supposed to give commencement "remarks" late in the ceremony, after remarks already delivered by the president, the student council president, the board president, and the president of the alumni council. I was pretty sure no one cared what I had to say by then, so I kept my speech as short as possible so we could get on with the reading of names and conferral of diplomas.

"Well, class of 2022, while I'm certain you have been anxiously awaiting a speech from the provost," (pause for polite laughter) "there is not much I can add to what others have so eloquently said here today. But there is one last opportunity I would like to offer you before you go, and that is the opportunity to thank your instructors. This group of accomplished scholars," with both arms I pointed toward the faculty, where they flanked the graduates in the center, "have gone through everything you've gone through in the past four years, while continuing to shepherd dozens or hundreds of young people through their classes to graduation. They've been available to you for advising, they've answered your late-night panic emails, they've learned how to use new technologies, they've helped you in your research and your labs and your performances and your writings and your creative endeavors." *Most of them, anyway.* "And, I might add, most of them have done it without the benefit and energy of youth!" (More genuine laughter.)

"I'm reminded of the saying that everything Fred Astaire did, Ginger Rogers did backwards and in high heels. So I invite you, the graduates, to join me in a round of applause for your faculty, who have danced tirelessly, backwards and in heels, to make you all look good these four years."

The student response was enthusiastic. They took to their feet immediately, whooping and hollering and clapping and waving to their favorites. The faculty looked gratified. I would keep looking for more ways to make their jobs better in the coming years. It was true what people said: teachers' teaching conditions are students' learning conditions. Anything I could do to improve life for the faculty was almost certain to make life better for their students, too.

It was finally time for Brody Aardsma to start the diploma line. Carefully I read 227 names according to the pronunciation notes I had been given. When Alyssa Zeggelink walked across the stage I breathed a sigh of relief. I had somehow made it through this crazy year.

After milling about outside the gym, schmoozing with parents, and congratulating faculty, I went back to my office to tie up loose ends. On my calendar was written "P?" I tried to remember what that was, annoyed with myself for leaving a cryptic reminder.

Then suddenly it came to me: today marked one full year since I got my last period. According to the experts, that meant I had crossed over from perimenopause into menopause. I stared at a shadow on the wall over my desk, trying and failing to figure out how I felt.

Just before six o'clock I packed up my briefcase and left the office. My left shoulder felt sore and I decided I would revert to carrying a backpack this summer. Who was I kidding with this "professional" style anyway? I missed my flannel shirts and leggings, and I was pretty sure a briefcase or lack of one wasn't going to ruin my administrative career.

It was sunny but, to my mind, freakishly cold for late May. I was mad at myself for not having worn the appropriate coat this morning, still getting used to this northern life. *Where's a good a hot flash when you need one?*

Upon approaching St. Margaret, I stopped. The sun was sinking directly behind her, giving her a shining halo, and pink crepuscular light draped across the campus around her. Having passed it a hundred times by now, I suddenly noticed the bush next to her was a lilac bush, at last in full bloom. I leaned in to smell it, and just as I did, a breeze caused a flowering tree overhead to start snowing tiny white petals into the air.

I watched in awe, feeling as if Margaret and I were two tiny figurines inside a snow globe. Time stopped. I breathed deeply. All seemed right with the world. *Are you there, Margaret? It's me, Jen. Thanks for watching out for me this year. I know I've been a bit of a wreck. I appreciate you sticking around so faithfully.*

My reverie was broken by a sky-ripping blast from a giant motorcycle with a helmetless rider. I turned furiously toward the sound and watched him ride away, still hearing him long after he was out of sight. *Asshole.*

When I turned back to St. Margaret, the patron saint of childbirth and pregnancy still looked down serenely, a lone petal resting on her left cheek. *Ok, fine, I suppose even he has a mother who loves him.* I checked to see if anyone was around. The coast seemed clear, so I tore off a single branch of lilac to take home.

As I neared the house, I saw Jamie on the sidewalk at the corner of Chapel and Birch, all six-foot-two of her, her fuzzy pink jacket blowing in the chilly breeze, walking toward me with her silly lopsided beast of a dog. Deirdre was sniffing around underneath another overgrown lilac bush that was threatening to take over the sidewalk.

I walked toward them and stopped. Jamie was wearing blue mascara and something shimmery on her cheekbones, so breathtakingly beautiful I wanted to kiss her. I suddenly felt a little bashful.

"Hello, darling," she said.

"I love you!" I declared out of nowhere. She burst out in a laugh that came all the way from down in her belly. I laughed too.

"I love you too!"

I was riding a wave. "I like, *love* love you."

"I *love* love you too," she said. Then we both stopped laughing and just smiled stupidly at each other. I felt my face grow hot. When I remembered to breathe, I broke the silence.

"Guess what."

"What?" she obliged.

"As of today, I have become a crone."

"You what?"

"I'm in menopause, officially. One year since my last period."

She gasped, eyes wide, the hint of a smile around her open mouth. She obviously took this as good news but wanted to make sure I thought so too. "How do you feel?"

"I don't know. Weird? Good."

"Weird and good," she repeated. "That sounds about right."

"Yep. Kind of like life." I leaned down and patted Deirdre, who was sniffing the toe of my boot. I couldn't wait to put slippers on.

"Should we celebrate?" she asked. "Or is that *too* weird?"

"Yeah!" I was flooded with gratitude to have made a new bosom friend in middle age. "I mean, no, it's not too weird. A little celebration sounds fun. A crone commencement. Like I'm...finally a real grown-up. Or something." That reminded me. "I should probably go say hello to my kids first."

"We can do it at your place," she offered. "I'll take Deirdre home and bring cocktails over in a little while."

"OK." I started to leave but then turned back. "Actually, why don't I take Deirdre now?" Jamie raised her eyebrows. "She should be allowed to visit our house. The kids love her, and Fiona can take care of herself. We could get a pizza and watch something stupid."

"Pizza and something stupid sounds perfect," she said with a smile.

Deirdre looked puzzled to be leaving with me, but after a longing glance toward Jamie she came along willingly. Walking her home, the word "perfect" bounced around my mind. Jamie's smile was perfect. Not having periods anymore was perfect. My kids being safe was perfect. The blooming lilacs were perfect. My thick legs walking me home were perfect.

I would be sweaty and cranky again soon enough. But for the moment—just that moment—I wouldn't change a thing.

Afterword: Journal of Met Needs

Hey, Margaret, there's no way I can possibly name every person who has meant something to me or met some of my needs during the writing of this novel. I love too many people to count—not because I am shallow, but because I am so damn lucky. I hope everyone I love knows I love them, so they don't need to be anxious about whether or not their names actually appear here. I am finishing this project in a hurry because I need to be done with it.

I wrote the first 50,000 words of *Midlife at St. Margaret's* during NaNoWriMo (National Novel Writing Month) 2021, not long after quitting my job as a professor. Regular online meet-ups with the Lansing NaNoWriMo group, led by Trish, were absolutely crucial to my start-up momentum. The idea for this book came from Angry.Sad.Motivated (@nlmtys, RIP Twitter), whose mid-pandemic tweet sent me back to the source. Judy Blume is a goddess, obviously.

Sherry Clark was an amazing and supportive editor, who helped me turn a first draft of my first novel manuscript into a much better manuscript, a version of which is now in your hands. Nothing you hate about this book should be blamed on Sherry. (And if you need an editor, you can find her on LinkedIn.) Kristi, Jess, Annie, Steven, Judith, and Charlie all read earlier drafts and offered encouragement and the odd editorial; Kristi even included it among her collections of book reviews on Facebook! So many other friends and family members shared their perimenopause experiences, asked me along the way how the novel was going, and generously didn't laugh at me for trying to write a novel. I so appreciate anyone, past or present, who takes the time to read this.

Chris, Gus, Watson, Cookie, JoJo, and Fleabag created the immediate cozy and nurturing backdrop of life that allowed me the time, space, and love required to finish a creative project I had always wondered if I could finish. My parents provided similar support from afar. I have no idea who I would be without them all.

And thanks to you, Margaret, for listening.